1976

F N   AY

INTERNATIONAL SERIES OF MONOGRAPHS IN
EXPERIMENTAL PSYCHOLOGY
GENERAL EDITOR: H. J. EYSENCK

Volume 6

RESEARCH AND EXPERIMENT
IN STUTTERING

Research and Experiment
in Stuttering

BY

H. R. BEECH, Ph.D.
Senior Lecturer in Psychology,
Institute of Psychiatry, University of London

AND

FAY FRANSELLA, Ph.D.
Research Associate, Mental Health Research Fund,
St. George's Hospital, University of London

PERGAMON PRESS

OXFORD · NEW YORK · TORONTO · SYDNEY · BRAUNSCHWEIG

Pergamon Press Ltd., Headington Hill Hall, Oxford
Pergamon Press Inc., Maxwell House, Fairview Park, Elmsford, New York 10523
Pergamon of Canada Ltd., 207 Queen's Quay West, Toronto 1
Pergamon Press (Aust.) Pty. Ltd., 19a Boundary St., Rushcutters Bay, N.S.W. 2011, Australia
Vieweg & Sohn GmbH, Burgplatz 1, Braunschweig

First edition 1968
Reprinted 1971

Library of Congress Catalog Card No. 68-18518

PRINTED IN GREAT BRITAIN BY A. WHEATON AND CO. LTD., EXETER
and reprinted lithographically by
COMPTON PRINTING LTD., LONDON AND AYLESBURY
08 012539 5

CONTENTS

v

LIST OF ILLUSTRATIONS

ACKNOWLEDGEMENT

The authors would like to express their thanks to Dr. Burl B. Gray for his comments and advice in the preparation of certain parts of this manuscript.

CHAPTER 1

THE BACKGROUND TO STUTTERING

1. *Introduction*

There are now available, in the form of books, monographs, and journal articles, many hundreds of contributions which are directly or indirectly concerned with the phenomena of stuttering. Much of this work is of a highly specialized and detailed character and may appear to have little to do with the most central and obtrusive characteristics of "stuttering" as the layman uses this term. Other work is of a more general character, particularly that concerning personality, but the impression gained by anyone surveying the literature on stuttering is that of the great diversity of interest and specialization which is involved; this impression may be especially surprising in terms of the superficial appearance of simplicity of stuttering as a disorder.

However, closer inspection of the stuttering field is revealing of complexities which have as yet failed to remit to the persistent efforts of research workers, and much experimental endeavour seems simply to raise new and more difficult problems. This latter observation is not unusual in any developing research area and might be regarded as evidence of progress in the sense that we are gradually learning which questions to ask and to recognize those issues which are of primary importance.

Nevertheless, part of the problem of conducting research and therapy in the field of stuttering may stem from the kinds of assumptions which are made *in advance of* experimental evidence. Perhaps the most obvious of these, and one which is undoubtedly easiest to make, is that stuttering is a unitary disorder and that stutterers belong to a particular class of individuals in a more fundamental sense than that they are all prone to experience difficulty in speaking. Usually this assumption is related to that of an "illness concept" of stuttering, in which the speech disturbance appears as a disease with its manifestations being regarded as symptoms.

In fact, as will be discussed in detail in the preliminary chapters of this book, stuttering can take many forms and may appear in many different psychological and physical settings, and there is, as yet, no hard evidence as to whether or not "stuttering" can be regarded as a unitary phenomenon. In view of this it is not surprising to find, as Chapter 2 indicates, that there is no general agreement on a definition of stuttering.

Problems exist, therefore, at the most basic level of description and we are still concerned with questions relating to what we mean by "stuttering" and how many different kinds of stuttering there might be.

Again, in terms of the explanatory frameworks, the situation is indicative of a primitive stage of development, with a rich crop of theories offering alternative accounts of a limited range of phenomena. While theories abound in the stuttering field it is generally agreed that none afford satisfactory explanation of the phenomena they set out to encompass. In this connection it is pertinent to point out that the adoption of certain theoretical positions to account for particular observations often seems to produce discrepant research findings.

Finally, as will be apparent from the material presented in this book, stuttering research is confounded and bedevilled by a lack of solid and reliable evidence, and an abundance of contradictory and conflicting experimental results.

To some extent the many divergent theoretical viewpoints and the lack of agreement on definition, as well as the great variety of methods of measurement and things measured, may have conspired to produce these effects; to some extent it may be that persistent, careful, co-ordinated and systematic research has been lacking in the field.

The chapters which follow are concerned with highlighting some of the problems which have arisen, whether these concern definition, measurement, theory, or conflicting evidence. However, in doing so it has not been our aim to provide a comprehensive account of all stuttering research, but rather to focus upon certain issues which are illustrative of problem areas in the field in general. This policy has naturally resulted in the omission of various important topics, notably that concerning treatment.

Respecting therapy, it seemed to us that so little detailed experimentation and research of a systematic character has been conducted that this particular area could be legitimately excluded from the book and, while therapeutic procedures are referred to from time to time, we have made no attempt to deal with them as a separate topic.

Again, because of our emphasis upon research and experiment, we have excluded reference to the more "notional" contributions to the field, particularly those involved in the psychoanalytic publications.

An attempt has been made to preserve some degree of logical relationship between the issues presented in any one chapter. Sometimes this has been a relatively simple matter, for example in the chapter concerning the stutterers' personality, but on occasions the logic may appear to be somewhat strained as in the case of the chapter dealing with Rhythm Effects, Delayed Auditory Feedback, and Operant Conditioning. It is hoped that this difficulty, where apparent, has not served to impair presentation and obscure important issues.

Finally, the authors felt that there was no place in a book of this kind for a separate chapter dealing with a summary of evidence presented and conclusions which might be drawn. To some extent the need for such an arrangement has been obviated by the inclusion of a summary of important points at the end of each chapter, but the main conclusions which can be drawn might be stated quite simply. First, it seems clear that the problems of aetiology and mechanisms of stuttering have not been resolved, nor are they likely to remit easily. Secondly, that there is an obvious need for considerably more agreement on the phenomena of stuttering and that classification, which is an important first step toward understanding, must be given more research attention.

Thirdly, while the volume of good research and experimentation shows signs of increasing, there is room for more concentrated, systematic, large-scale projects if significant advances in the field are to be made.

Before introducing the problems referred to in detail the authors considered that some attention should be given to certain background information. Accordingly we have, in the next section of this chapter, made reference to several matters including sex ratios of stutterers, incidence of stuttering, and prognosis of the disorder. These matters, it is hoped, might provide a broad basis or background in terms of which material presented in later chapters might be evaluated.

2. *The Manifestations of Stuttering*

The term "stuttering" usually refers to particular forms of interruption to the free flow of speech with sufficient frequency to significantly impede verbal communication. Typically it is assumed that there exists no actual mechanical impairment to the organs of speech (of tongue, palate, etc.) and that, as these vocal mechanisms are intact, the cause or causes of the disorder must be sought in terms of "higher order" functions of either a psychological or neurophysiological kind, or both. However, the absence of conclusive evidence concerning the mechanisms which may be involved and responsible for stuttering phenomena leads inevitably to an emphasis in diagnosis upon the *overt* expressions or "symptoms" of the disorder(s). Consequently diagnostic considerations tend to be exclusively concerned with the manifestations of stuttering which might be observed by anyone listening to the speech of affected persons, or able to make visual observations of the struggle to achieve communication. Relatively little difficulty might be expected in drawing diagnostic conclusions, especially in the case of severe stuttering, and most published papers show no concern with the problems of identification of members of this group, usually confining classificatory considerations to those involving the degree of severity of the speech difficulty. On the other hand, it could be argued that diagnostic refinements might, at least on occasions, be of considerable importance in view of the range and complexity of difficulties which have been associated with the disorder(s).

It is interesting, in this connection, to note a study by Barr (1940) which, while only employing a small group of 10 subjects, gives some indication of the range of phenomena which are often considered in attaching the diagnostic label "stutterer". In this study subjects were asked to read material aloud while two observers and certain mechanical devices recorded the appearance of various abnormalities, including those having to do with sound production, breathing, the musculature of voice production and face, as well as general postural changes. Altogether twenty-five specific phenomena were observed among the group members, such as movements of the forehead, jaw-tremor, breath-holding, prolongation of sounds, etc., but it was noted that certain of these features were to be more commonly observed than were others, and also that the number, pattern, and significance of these specific phenomena varied from individual to individual.

Studies like that of Barr serve to remind us that any narrow view of stuttering manifestations being confined to a difficulty in speech production might be misleading. Obviously, while difficulty in verbal communication is of central importance "stuttering", as a diagnostic classification, typically carries implications of numerous additional abnormalities and the total pattern and significance of these abnormalities may be of great interest.

One of the earliest and most obvious characteristics is the tendency for repetitions, especially of syllables, to occur. Repetitions of phrases, words, and syllables are common among very young children and are not usually regarded as indicative of stuttering. Métraux (1950), for example, reports that 23 children aged 18 months showed easy and unforced repetition which could be easily terminated by the child itself or by others, while at 2 years a type of compulsive repetition of word or phrase can be observed, and by the age of $4\frac{1}{2}$ years repetitions are seldom found. Similarly, Davis (1939) has described repetitions as being part of the speech pattern of children up to 5 years of age, with syllable repetitions being more common among boys than girls. The diagnosis of stuttering tends to be made when repetitions continue to occur with a statistically greater frequency than would ordinarily be expected at a particular age level. However, it must be obvious that conclusions in this respect are ordinarily drawn by a child's parents or guardians without recourse to refined observation, measurement, and knowledge of the available evidence, so that assessment in this particular is often non-rigorous.

Johnson's theory, which will be discussed in greater detail in a later section, argues that this point is perhaps crucial in determining whether the "normal" disfluency of a young child will become a stutter, and this view is supported by fairly strong evidence. It is indeed difficult to see, for example, how the disfluencies of a 2-year-old can be identified as stuttering excepting in terms of stringent and exaggerated standards of fluency which may be imposed by parents, and it is of interest to note that in the study reported by Andrews and Harris (1964) 8 % of the sample were said to have experienced the onset of stuttering at this age. Pointing up the importance of this statistic is the further observation from this study that repetitions were regarded as being associated with the onset of stuttering in 92 % of the cases considered.

Nevertheless, repetition of word sounds, most typically *initial* word sounds, is one of the most common and obtrusive of stuttering phenomena, and is likely to excite the attention of the listener, especially if several repetitions of the same speech sound occur in succession.

It is argued, however, that while the *frequency* with which repetitions mark the speech of stutterers is an important feature, the *tension* which may accompany this aspect of the disturbance is also diagnostic. Manifestations of psychological and physical tension certainly appear to serve to differentiate the "normal" repetitions of the young child from those of the mature speaker with a stutter, and it is often said that such tension arises out of the attention which parents and others might pay to early examples of nonfluency. It is, therefore, not surprising that many therapists have attached considerable importance to dealing with tension states associated with stuttering, especially as such states may involve the whole body and are not necessarily confined to speech and respiratory musculature. Bender (1935) has, for example, advocated special exercises and participation in physical activities with the purpose of encouraging the relaxation of important muscle groups.

In this connection Hollingsworth (1939) has carried out an interesting investigation of the ways in which chewing gum might reduce tension, and has concluded that this activity might have some therapeutic value. In this study "nervous restlessness" (any motor activity irrelevant to the task) and feelings of "strain" and muscle tension, were reduced by from 5 to 15% in a group of 20 subjects.

Just how physical exercise or relaxation procedures help in the modification of stuttering is not known, but at least two possibilities suggest themselves; either the amount of effort which is put into speech activity is being diminished substantially, or some form of training in the selective control of musculature is being acquired. Whether either of these general formulations is correct, or whether other mechanisms are responsible, must remain the subject of further research.

Other workers in the field appear to place greater emphasis upon *psychological* rather than *physical* tensions. Usually the former are seen as arising out of emotional maladjustments which go deeper than those which might accrue from the immediacy of the situation of being unable to communicate fluently (e.g. Honig, 1947; Glauber, 1958). Typically, those concerned with tensions sponsored by emotional problems tend to adopt a psychodynamic frame of reference and are relatively unconcerned with the experimental approach which forms the subject matter of this book.

A further important diagnostic feature of stuttering is the tendency for prolongations of sounds to occur, where the utterance of the sound, especially of vowels, is drawn out for an appreciably longer period of time than is characteristic of nonstutterers. Indeed, sound prolongation is an important feature of this type of speech disorder in that it is rarely found in the speech of normally fluent individuals.

In Voelker's study (1944) 62 nonstuttering orphans and 7 stutterers were required to speak for 5 minutes and the speech errors and difficulties were noted. It is of interest to note that while hesitancies and repetitions occurred in both groups—stutterers being differentiated simply in terms of the frequency with which those manifestations occurred—prolongations appeared to be peculiar to the stutterers and hence assume special diagnostic significance.

Prolongation of spoken sounds, so far as can be determined, appears to occur later in the developmental sequence of stuttering and may, in consequence, not be regarded as included in any definition of "Primary Stuttering". However, a study by Glasner and Vermilyea (1953) suggests that a substantial percentage of speech and hearing specialists (19%) may regard prolongations as part of "Primary Stuttering" although the term itself, as this study suggests, tends to have different connotations for different people some of whom regard the term as of little or no value, or use it as a description of normal disfluencies, or in connection with the presence or absence of *awareness* of speech difficulty.

While prolongations are certainly very common and obtrusive among stutterers, and are of considerable diagnostic significance because of the infrequency with which they occur among normally fluent individuals, it is of some interest that the latter group are prone to manifest this type of speech response under conditions of delayed auditory feedback (D.A.F.). This observation may in fact suggest that the speech disturbances produced by D.A.F. conditions are unlike those *initially* found among so-called stutterers (i.e. hesitancies and repetitions), and that the mechanisms involved in the production of prolongations by D.A.F. and in stuttering are different. Whatever relation exists between prolongations of speech sounds in stuttering and those effected by D.A.F. it is interesting to note, in this connection, that Goldiamond (1965) has observed that this abnormality might be usefully encouraged and developed among stutterers owing to its susceptibility to "shaping" into normal speech patterns by means of operant conditioning procedures. A more detailed discussion of D.A.F. will be presented in a later section of this book.

A fourth feature of stuttering, and one which is characteristically very distressing for both the speaker and the listener, concerns the silent blocks during which the former appears to be unable to produce any vocalization at all in spite of strenuous efforts. This phenomenon is often obtrusive among stutterers and provides a good measure of speech difficulty in view of the ease with which the *latency* of speech, following presentation of some stimulus word, can be assessed. This measure has, for example, been employed in a study by Beech and Fransella (1966) which is reported in the section concerning the control of stuttering by rhythm. Such blocks, like other characteristics of stuttering, are most frequently observed in connection with the initiation of words, phrases, or sentences, and it is not surprising that this phenomenon has stimulated some degree of interest in the breathing of stutterers. The "breathing symptoms" of stutterers have been studied by Steer (1937), among others, who investigated differences in this variable between 67 stutterers and 20 fluent children. However, in this study no differences between the two groups were observed on the various measures of breathing function employed.

An earlier attempt to investigate the breathing of stutterers was carried out by Fossler (1930), who obtained records from both experimental (stuttering) and control (fluent) groups. In this study it was found that while the *volume* of inspiration and expiration did not differentiate the groups the stutterers showed considerably greater *variability* in their patterns of inspiration and expiration. It was also observed that the experimental group tended to show marked individual differences in their respiratory patterns. It is interesting to note that Murray (1932) was able to confirm the finding of great variability in breathing responses among stutterers.

Van Riper (1936) has also reported upon certain breathing characteristics of stutterers, and he states that this group tends to be characterized by consistent forms of thoracic breathing during a block in the flow of speech.

More recently, Starbuck and Steer (1954) have carried out an investigation of both thoracic and abdominal breathing in stutterers, using 22 experimental subjects and the same number of relevantly matched controls who were fluent speakers. It was found that the former group showed both a reduction in the number of complete thoracic and abdominal breathing cycles on repeated reading of a 200-word prose passage.

The evidence in general, therefore, suggests that differences in the patterning of respiratory responses exist between normally fluent persons and stutterers, and it seems likely that the "blocks" which stutterers experience are associated with such responses. Whether abnormalities of breathing are productive of blocks, or are the result of blocks occurring is not known, although it might be guessed from indirect evidence that the latter alternative is the more probable.

Also obtrusive among the features of stuttering are the peculiarities and abnormalities of motor activity which often seem to be as troublesome to the stutterer as the speech difficulty itself. Such activity is not confined to the musculature of jaws, tongue, etc., but may involve the facial muscles, trunk and limbs of the individual in exaggerated and irrelevant movement. This motor disturbance, when it occurs, is typically associated with moments of speech difficulty and both stutterers and therapists are inclined to regard the former as secondary and as arising out of strenuous attempts to overcome nonfluency by muscular effort.

It is usually argued that while the vigorous motor activity is un-successful in securing release from a block, such activity becomes inevitably *associated* with release by virtue of its temporal position in the block-release sequence, and is therefore likely to become a fixed and permanent part of the stuttering complex. In other words, when the speech block occurs the stutterer adopts certain strategies to effect release, among which often occurs pronounced muscular effort. At some stage fluent speech is resumed (differences in opinion exist concerning how fluency is achieved) and a connection is per-ceived, by the stutterer, between the preceding motor activity and the occurrence of fluency. This connection, once perceived, rapidly becomes firmly fixed,, the "validity" of the causal link being con-stantly endorsed by the invariable temporal sequence of motor activity being followed by cessation of stuttering. At some stage, however, it may well appear that the stutterer has lost his voluntary control over the motor activity which was designed and adapted to help in overcoming his speech disorder.

Some idea of the seriousness of this problem might be obtained from Bloodstein's study (1960a,b, 1961) involving over 400 children. He reports that the percentage of children in his sample manifesting motor symptomatology associated with stuttering appears to be a function of age, reaching a figure of about 70% among older sufferers. This finding not only points to the seriousness of the symptom in terms of its prevalence, but tends to endorse the view that the phenomenon is probably secondary in character. Bloodstein's findings also indicate that, among the range of motor abnormalities, those movements which involve the face and the respiratory system are quite common, while those which involve the trunk and limbs are comparatively infrequently found.

In view of these observations concerning the motor symptoma-tology of stutterers it is not surprising to find that many therapists raise strong objections to any treatment which might involve pro-viding the stutterer with new and more elaborate motor responses. The fear exists that while such responses may initially assist in the production of fluent speech, by "distraction" or some other mechan-ism, there is a tendency for such devices to become ineffective in their control of speech abnormalities and to remain as part of a growing repertoire of redundant motor activity.

A further problem area in the characteristics of the stutterer might be called "avoidance behaviour". This characteristic, when it appears, may seem to represent the stutterer's acceptance of his lack of fluency and probably reflects his striving to avoid the unpleasant consequences of nonfluency, both in terms of the impact on his own self-esteem and the effect upon the listener. Avoidance may take many forms but two broad classes of this tendency might be usefully distinguished; first, the avoidance of *specific stimuli* which are associated with speech difficulty, e.g. particular letters, sounds, or words, and secondly, avoidance of *situations* in which the specific stimuli associated with stuttering are likely to occur.

Bloodstein, in the studies referred to above, has pointed out that "difficult" words may be avoided by circumlocution or by the use of synonyms, although such tactics are obviously more readily available to older persons and are consequently more often observed among later age groups.

However, one of the problems facing the stutterer in making use of avoidance practices is the apparent susceptibility to generalization or spread of the difficulty so that, for example, the synonym newly adopted may quickly acquire some of the properties of the word originally avoided. This outcome would, in the case of the example quoted, be made more likely if the avoidance were mainly concerned with the *meaning* of a word rather than its specific alphabetical form.

Avoidance of situations which expose the stutterer to public display of his nonfluency, or in which he is likely to experience unusual difficulty, is understandable. It is, therefore, not remarkable to find that some stutterers tend to develop a rather unique existence for themselves which excludes their participation in many ordinary and everyday activities. This has led some therapists to emphasize the importance of the stutterer's possible "resistance" to any form of treatment, as any "cure" must inevitably involve a fairly radical and profound readjustment of personal life, including attitudes, standards, values, and behaviour.

An interesting attempt to classify and describe the implications of avoidance behaviour among stutterers was made by Kimmell (1938). This study involved the examination of twenty-nine autobiographical accounts written by stutterers, which were rated independently by two judges in terms of whether or not the avoidance had affected certain aspects of adjustment. It was concluded that stuttering avoidance reactions can operate so as to severely restrict the individual's development and range of social experience, as such reactions are found in the home, school, and other settings. The net effect appears to be that more time is spent in isolation from others, and, in addition, the type of job one does, the activities in which one engages, and relationships with other people all require more careful consideration and present more limited opportunities for the stutterer than for the fluent person. Until one gives careful attention to the problems of the stutterer, it is easy to overlook the degree of dependence upon verbal communication which is necessary to adequate functioning, and it is entirely reasonable to expect that some degree of maladjustment might arise from the avoidance activities found among some members of this group.

The development of a stutter is usually seen, therefore, to pass through various stages, from the simple repetition of sounds and words, through the exacerbation of prolongations and "blocking", and then to the development of disturbances of motor activity, leading ultimately in some individuals to avoidance activities, emotional disturbances, and other forms of social and psychological disruption. It is, of course, important to point out that not all stutterers pass through these stages, and may not do so in the order presented above, but it can be argued that this pattern might be regarded as representative of the phases in the development of a severe stutter. On other occasions, for other individuals, a mild degree of hesitancy, blocking, or repetitive speech may be the only manifestations of speech difficulty.

3. The Incidence and Prevalence of Stuttering

Most authorities are in agreement that stuttering is probably a function of many different kinds of variables and any answer to the question of incidence may have little real meaning except to indicate the magnitude of the problem to be dealt with. In addition, the question of incidence has usually been raised in connection with certain prescribed geographical locations, but such figures may not be a true representation of total stuttering incidence on a wider basis, e.g. certain cultures are said to be free of stuttering (Stewart, 1960), while others are alleged to have a characteristically high figure (Lemert, 1953). In general it would appear that few studies provide adequate information upon which to base a calculation as to the incidence of stuttering, and such studies tend to refer to either British or American samples. Even among the relatively better studies of stuttering incidence the methods of collecting and recording information, as well as sampling considerations, are far from satisfactory.

One study carried out, which gives some idea of stuttering incidence in Britain, has been reported by Spence et al. (1954), Morley, (1957), and Miller et al. (1960). For children up to age 7, almost 4% of the sample of 1000 children showed stuttering or speech hesitancy. According to Andrews and Harris (1964), it was later calculated that approximately 3% of the total group were stutterers or had stuttered for 6 months or longer by the time they were 16 years of age, and if 16 "transient" stutterers were to be included, then the "true" incidence among the 1000 children would be 4·5%.

Andrews and Harris (1964) also report the results of an inquiry involving 206 adults attending their general practitioners, who were asked about the occurrence of stuttering in their families. Ten of the 206 gave a personal history of stuttering, while 22 of the 615 family members of these patients were said to be, or to have been, stutterers. Thus, 4·8% of the interviewees were or had been stutterers, and 3·6% of the families of interviewees were similarly classified.

Andrews and Harris also obtained lists, compiled by teachers, of all children who stuttered in schools within the boundaries of the City of Newcastle upon Tyne. Teachers were provided with a brief description of the phenomenon they were to diagnose and the authors claim that no stutterers were overlooked, although there are no obvious reasons for believing this claim to be beyond doubt. Of the total school population aged 9–11 years surveyed (7358 children), the number of stutterers reported was 86, representing a figure of just over 1 %. This figure is very close to that found in other studies representing the incidence of *persistent* stuttering, and the rate is, of course, lower than that found at particular age levels below about 10 years as this will include those having transient stutters.

In spite of obvious sampling limitations, a study by Heltman (1940) also arrived at incidence figures around the 1 % mark. Of nearly 1600 new admissions to Syracuse University examined by Heltman, 20 stutterers were found, representing an incidence of 1·3 %.

A comprehensive study of stuttering among school-children has also been conducted by McDowell (1928). A survey of a cross-section of New York schools, involving a population of over 7000 children, produced a total of 61 stutterers, suggesting an incidence among school-children of less than 1 %. This figure is perhaps a little less than might be expected on the basis of other results obtained from samples of children.

A similar study was carried out by Travis *et al.* (1937), but also suffered from sampling limitations arising out of the main purpose of the inquiry—which was to investigate the influence of bilingualism upon stuttering. Some 4827 children, aged 4–17 years, were surveyed and 126 were found to stutter, indicating an incidence of 2·6 %. A comparison of the occurrence of stuttering among English speakers only and those children speaking both English and some other language revealed that the respective percentages were 1·80 and 2·80.

Morgenstern's (1956) survey of the relation between socio-economic factors and stuttering also contains useful information concerning the incidence of the disorder. Of nearly 30,000 10–11-year-old children who formed part of the survey, 350 were judged to be stutterers, representing a figure of approximately 1–2 %. This figure might be assumed to be just a little higher than the prevalence figure for the population as a whole which is probably about 1 %.

An interesting aspect of the expected incidence of stuttering is contained in a report by Berry (1938) who examined data collected from 250 parents of twins. In this survey, instead of stuttering incidence running at the usual 1%, the figure was a little more than 5% among all the siblings of twinning families.

Appropriate figures for the prevalence of stuttering among total populations are not available.

4. *The Prognosis for Stutterers*

References to partially successful treatments or complete cures for stuttering appear frequently in the literature, the surprising feature of these claims being that they derive from apparently very different forms of therapy and often involve dissimilar theoretical positions. Hogewind (1940), for example, has reported that improvement accompanies the administration of a vagal sedative, while Hale (1951) has suggested that a course of thiamin (vitamin B) has resulted in clear improvement of speech disturbances in 55% of stutterers. Other studies have suggested that beneficial results can be obtained from E.C.T. (Owen and Stemmermann, 1947), negative practice (Fishman, 1937), non-reinforcement (Sheehan, 1951), negative reinforcement (Goldiamond, 1965), psychoanalysis (Glauber, 1958), rhythmical speech (Meyer and Mair, 1963), chewing therapy (Kastein, 1947), "ventriloquism" (Froeschels, 1950), psychodrama (Lemert and Van Riper, 1944), hypnosis (Moore, 1946), syllable-timed speech (Andrews and Harris, 1964), and various other procedures, both physical and psychological. This massive array of "helpful" therapeutic techniques may serve to encourage the stutterer that one or other may assist him, but it should also serve to excite some alarm among practitioners and theorists concerned with stuttering phenomena. The situation should convey to most people the clear message that no obviously satisfactory treatment for stuttering is yet available.

Prognosis must inevitably be linked with treatment, at least for those suffering from severe stutters, but it is impossible at this stage to offer any reasonable guide as to which form of therapy is likely to prove helpful. It may be, of course, that different treatments are necessary for different cases and that any view of stuttering as a single disease entity is grossly misleading; or it could be that, typically, stuttering is a compound of many different and independent difficulties each of which must be the subject of a separate therapeutic attack. What seems to be the case at this stage is that no single or multiple form of treatment is characterized by more than a modest degree of success. The situation, in this respect, has remained static since Bryngelson's (1935) statement that an absolute cure for the adult stutterer is very rare indeed.

Bryngelson properly regards the issue of prognosis as being quite different for adults and children, remarking that some 40% of children will "lose" their speech handicap before the age of 8 years, presumably without any form of treatment at all.

According to Bryngelson the prognosis for adult stutterers is more hopeful if he is sufficiently intelligent to appreciate the therapeutic goals and procedures, is determined, possesses the necessary self-discipline to carry out his therapeutic assignments, and has a satisfactory environment. Young stutterers, on the other hand, are said to have a better prognosis as one has often to deal only with the "primary neurologic spasm" uncomplicated by the secondary elaborations of speech difficulty and emotional problems which beset the adult stutterer of long standing.

However, the features to which Bryngelson refers as indicative of good prognosis must be regarded as only tentative, and the generalizations which can be made about recovery of fluency are few. Perhaps the only statistic in this respect in which one might have reasonable confidence is that relating to the spontaneous remission of stuttering among children, which indicates that while approximately 3–5% of the total population may experience an episode of stuttering in childhood, the persistence of the disorder arises only among about 1%. Of these persistent stutterers some will recover, but no precise figures are available for this group, and any attempt to estimate this proportion from a survey of the literature is likely to be misleading as a tendency to relapse is commonly reported.

5. *The Relation between Age and Stuttering*

The influence of age upon patterns of speech is of obvious importance from both a theoretical and a practical standpoint, and it is understandable that much controversy centres around the age factor in this field. The weight of evidence suggests that stuttering has its "true" onset early in life, typically before the age of 8 years, and that later onset—particularly the development of a stutter in adulthood—is comparatively rare.

So far as can be determined, the first appearance of stuttering in later life tends to be associated with, or precipitated by, sudden and intense physical or psychological stresses. For example, Arend *et al.* (1962) have reported the occurrence of such disturbance as the result of brain damage, and Peacher and Harris (1946) have related the onset of stuttering to the psychological trauma of wartime experiences. However, interest has centred upon the early years of life as important in the development of this form of speech disturbance simply because of the statistical frequency with which its occurrence has been observed in young children.

Certain theories of stuttering take the view that the disorder arises quite "naturally" out of the kind of disfluencies which are characteristically found among normal children and that age, as a factor, is of interest simply as affording a basis for learning to perpetuate existing speech patterns. In this event it is clear that the developmental aspects of speech are of obvious interest to those holding this view of stuttering aetiology, and the results of studies by Davis (1939, 1940a, b) assume considerable importance.

In one study (1939) Davis examined the speech of 62 boys and girls ranging in age from 2 to 5 years. She found considerable variability between children in the number of repetitions, but noted that phrase repetition was most common, followed by word repetition, while syllable repetition was least frequently observed. Repetition was in fact very common indeed in this group, the repetition of one word in every four uttered being regarded as quite normal. As Davis's group ranged in intelligence from "average" to "superior" it seems quite possible that repetitions could be even more frequent than her figures indicate.

A further interesting feature of this inquiry was that while phrase and word repetition shared a tendency to decrease with age this was not the case for syllable repetition which remained at the same level. Furthermore, it seemed that those who appeared to be deviant from the group in terms of speech behaviour were those in whom syllable repetition tended to be high.

In her second paper Davis (1940a) reports the results of correlating the observed forms of repetition with measures of language maturity. In this study none of the correlations were found to be sufficiently high to provide a satisfactory explanation of repetitive speech.

While these findings afford some degree of support for those claiming that stuttering arises (e.g. through differential reinforcement) out of "normal" disfluencies, the evidence is obviously not conclusive. The main contention of those who might oppose this hypothesized link between stuttering and normal speech would be that syllable repetition is the least common form and that one might reasonably have expected stuttering to involve word or phrase repetition if the disorder represented the elaboration and prolongation of "normal" disfluencies.

Similarly, a study reported by Steer (1937) is of importance. This investigation, involving 67 stutterers aged 3–13 years, and 20 fluent children aged 3–5 years, set out to test the validity of the assumption that certain features of stuttering could be observed regardless of age or developmental level. Using measures of both "vocal" and "breathing" characteristics, the author concluded that one or all of three propositions might be true. First, that children do not stutter, but some of them evidence deviations with greater frequency than others; secondly, that most children stutter, and that the persistence of this pattern of symptoms occurs among some people; thirdly, that the features which are generally held to indicate "stuttering" do not differentiate stutterers from nonstutterers at the pre-school level.

A later study with similar aims to those described by Davis was carried out by Métraux (1950). Observations were made of the speech patterns of 207 children ranging from 18 months to 54 months of age. The results again indicate that repetition is very common among normal children, and that it shows some variation in kind as well as in frequency at particular age levels. At 18 months of age repetition is "easy and unforced" and is very frequent; several months later a more compulsive form of repetition is observed, but by the age of 4 years repetitions are much less prominent.

The difficult problem, of course, is that of differentiating "normal" speech difficulties from stuttering; this differentiation would be clearly hazardous at an early age, yet it is possible that the speech patterns which are characteristic of the potential stutterer are recognizable and distinguishable from the beginnings of speech. On the other hand, Johnson, as will be discussed in detail later in this book, thinks it likely that stuttering only emerges out of the recognition and labelling of normal fluencies as "stutters" and that, at early stages of speech development, no differences in speech patterns exist between those who will and those who will not be afflicted. In his paper Johnson (1942) concluded that in 92% of cases of stuttering the phenomena which were diagnosed as stuttering were the *effortless* repetitions of sounds, phrases, words, and syllables.

Should Johnson's view be correct then some doubt may be cast upon investigations which locate the onset in stuttering as being during the very early years of a child's development. How much credence can be attached, for example, to Berry's (1932) findings which indicate the average age of onset of stuttering to be 4·86 years? While this study was broadly based and comprised some 430 medical records of stutterers and 462 records of nonstutterers, the quality of the evidence might be questioned especially in view of the evidence presented from studies such as that carried out by Bloodstein et al. (1952).* In this study 48 parents were asked to judge whether a child was a stutterer or a normal speaker after listening to recorded speech samples of "stuttering" and nonstuttering children aged 3½–10 years. It was observed that parents of "stutterers" were significantly more likely to judge a child to be a stutterer regardless of whether the child had been or had not been labelled as such.

Several studies have, however, suggested that differences between the early speech patterns of stutterers and nonstutterers are observable. In one such investigation, Glasner (1949) concludes that the repetitions of these two groups can be distinguished, although this evidence emphasized qualitative rather than quantitative aspects of the disturbance.

Again, other studies have implicated age in a different way as an important factor in nonfluency. One study by Morley (1957), for example, suggests that the development of speech is delayed in stutterers and that when speech makes its appearance it is more likely to be accompanied by some defect of articulation. Similar results to those quoted by Morley have also been reported by Berry and Eisenson (1956) and indicate that certain evidence points to the delayed onset and development of speech among stutterers.

A recent study by Spence et al. (1954) suggests that the prevalence of stuttering shows some degree of variability with age, with an increase up to the age of 8 years, and then a decrease thereafter until the prevalence figure reaches approximately 1%. The onset of stuttering after age 11 was not noted, and this investigation thus endorses that of others in finding that if stuttering has not occurred by puberty then the likelihood of developing this form of speech abnormality is negligible.

The study by Andrews and Harris (1964) is of considerable interest in this respect, although the information upon which their figures are based does not inspire great confidence, for example

* However, see Chapter 2, p. 38.

assessment of the child's speech at school and at the clinic, and the "mother's remembered history of events". The two interesting features of their findings in respect of age of onset of stuttering; first that of the 80 stutterers considered (aged 9–11 years at the time of the inquiry), 95% had commenced to stutter by the age of 7, and all had developed the disorder by the age of 9. A more detailed account of the relationship between age and stuttering onset reported by Andrews and Harris is shown in Fig. 1.

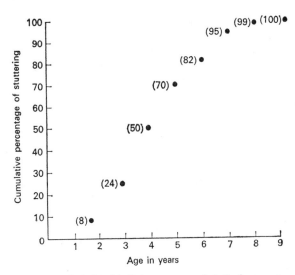

FIG. 1. Relationship between age and stuttering onset.

While the diagnosis of stuttering at the age of 2 years might appear suspect, these findings appear to be similar to those reported by others. Morley (1957), for example, in a review of 400 clinic cases of stuttering, found that 50% had shown evidence of the disorder before the age of 5 years, and that almost all cases showed onset before the age of 13.

The second interesting feature concerning age of onset of stuttering in the Harris and Andrews study, is that relating the onset to severity of the symptoms. Their data suggest that in some 70% of children characterized by a "moderate or severe" stutter the symptoms had appeared before the age of 5 years, 33% showing evidence of some defect with the onset of speech. On the other hand, of the 56 cases of "mild stuttering", only 9% had evidenced some signs of the disturbance with the onset of speech.

In summary, the evidence respecting age and stuttering is equivocal, some data suggesting that differences in fluency *are* apparent during the early years of the child's life, while other data purport to show that no such differentiation is possible. On the whole the available information is weighted in favour of there being observable differences which are independent of "labelling" by parents or other authorities, but firm conclusions cannot be drawn until more detailed, searching and well-controlled inquiries have been made.

6. *The Relation between I.Q. and Stuttering*

Frequent reference is made to observations that stutterers tend to be more intelligent than average, for example Stein (1942) accepts this observation as well documented and appears to attribute it to a greater "richness of imagination" producing an interference between ideas which "jostle one another" in seeking vocalization. However, much of the evidence which has been quoted is anecdotal in character, and firm conclusions concerning the relation between stuttering and intelligence must be drawn on the basis of hard empirical evidence rather than opinion.

It is not entirely clear why one should expect to find differences between stutterers and nonstutterers in terms of level of cognitive functioning and it would seem that, more often than not, such differences as have been apparent in any particular study have been interpreted on a *post-hoc* basis. It might, however, be tentatively suggested that should stuttering be shown to have an "organic" basis it would be more probable that stutterers would be characterized by some form of general or specific cognitive defect; the argument that stuttering is associated with higher levels of intelligence would be somewhat weaker and involve the kind of conceptions put forward by Stein and referred to above.

One of the earliest studies in this area was carried out by McDowell (1928) who set out to compare stutterers and nonstutterers in terms of both intelligence and school achievement. A survey of an economic and social cross-section of New York schools was conducted and 61 stutterers were found, boys in the sample outnumbering girls by about 3 to 1. The stutterers were reported as having Stanford-Binet I.Q.s ranging from 63 to 156, with the average I.Q. being 99·14. If one can assume that the sampling was reasonably representative of the population at large, then it would appear that the results of this study reflect no differences between stutterers and nonstutterers in cognitive functioning. The educational achievement scores on tests of arithmetic, reading, and spelling also failed to produce evidence of poorer performance among stutterers, the achievement quotient of the group being 100. Furthermore, tests of vocabulary and fluency (measured in terms of the number of words produced within a 3-minute period) taken from the Binet also failed to differentiate the stutterers from a matched control group, suggesting that a specific impairment of language ability in stutterers is unlikely.

A study by Davis (1940a, b) also appears to afford some degree of indirect confirmation of McDowell's findings. Here, in a study of 62 pre-school children, it was found that repetitions had only a slight negative relationship with I.Q.

On the other hand, Travis (1959) has reported that the average intelligence of a group of 73 child stutterers was significantly better than normal, while Schindler (Johnson, 1955) found stutterers to be slightly below the average in respect of intelligence.

One of the most recent studies in which the intelligence of stutterers was assessed is that carried out by Andrews and Harris (1964). Their study, involving 80 stutterers and 80 control children, indicated that the groups were significantly differentiated on the Wechsler Intelligence Scale for Children, although the absolute difference was not large, stutterers having a full scale I.Q. of 94·7 and nonstutterers one of 101·8. A further interesting feature of this inquiry concerns the finding that, contrary to what might have been expected, there was no significant discrepancy between the scores of stutterers on the verbal and performance scales of the W.I.S.C.

Some degree of attention has been paid to the frequency of occurrence of speech difficulties among children of subnormal intelligence, and the outcome strongly suggests that stuttering is found significantly more frequently among this group than among children of normal intelligence. In one early study Loutit and Halls (1936) observed that the prevalence of stuttering among E.S.N. children was more than three times as great as that found in normals. An even higher prevalence among subnormals was reported by Schlanger and Gottsleben (1957) who examined the speech of over

500 defectives with an average I.Q. of 50. The prevalence in this study was observed to be 17%, which contrasts sharply with the figure usually found among samples of normal children.

Other studies (e.g. Wohl 1951) also endorse the greater frequency of occurrence of stuttering among children of low intelligence.

While the difficulties of assessment must play some part in determining the different figures for incidence among subnormals, the consistency of the finding strongly suggests that, at lower levels of intelligence, the occurrence of stuttering and intelligence are in some way associated. To some extent the presence of organic factors may be implicated as a common factor producing both intellectual deficit and speech disturbance, but it may also be that more "psychological" factors are involved, for example the absence of environmental influences which might help in overcoming "normal" disfluencies.

In summary it might be said that, within the normal ranges of intelligence, there are probably no observable differences in the level of cognitive functioning, either of a general or a specific type. On the other hand, among the intellectually subnormal, stuttering certainly appears to be more prevalent, although the influences which contribute to this association are at present unknown.

7. *The Relationship of Stuttering to Sex*

Perhaps one of the most outstanding findings in stuttering research is that concerning the higher incidence of stuttering among males. While the quoted sex ratio for stuttering shows some variation from study to study, the observation that stuttering is more common among males is remarkably consistent. It is not surprising, therefore, that this link between sex and stuttering has constituted one of the basic "facts" which the theorist attempts to incorporate in his model with a greater or lesser degree of success.

In essence two quite different theoretical accounts of this phenomenon have been put forward. The first argues that there are differences in the physical make-up of the sexes (e.g. in metabolism), which are inherited or part of the individual's constitution, rendering males more susceptible to development of speech disturbance. The main alternative view is that the psychological environment for boys and girls—at least in "Western" society—is typically quite different, boys being placed under considerably greater stress in terms of demands made upon them, and this imposed strain makes stuttering more probable among males. Sometimes "mixed" theories are put forward which incorporate both "physical" and psychological factors, for example that the stresses of growing up are "felt" more by boys than by girls because the latter have a much more rapid maturational development.

McDowell's (1928) survey of New York City schools involved some 7000 children, of whom 61 were found to be stutterers. The ratio of male to female stutterers in this investigation was found to be 2·9:1. These figures were confirmed by Schindler (Johnson, 1955) who reported the proportion of male to female stutterers to be 3:1.

Rather higher ratios have been found by other investigators, for example Morley (1952) found that males were four times as frequently seen in the clinic as were girls for the treatment of stuttering, and Wepman (1939) reported the same ratio in his investigation employing 250 stutterers and 250 fluent subjects. On the other hand, lower ratios have been observed, for example Spence *et al.* (1954) found, during a large-scale inquiry which resulted in the discovery of 27 stutterers, that stuttering was 2·4 times more common among males than females.

Reid (1946) has quoted reported male/female stuttering ratios ranging from 2:1 up to as much as 10:1, and Schuell (1946) has recorded reports of similar discrepancies. The ratio of males to females varies with the age band under consideration, and the variety of prevalence ratios quoted may, to some degree, reflect the influence of this variable. What evidence is available in this connection suggests that the prevalence of stuttering in males and females becomes more disparate as age increases, and one possible explanation of this could be that while girls and boys are equally susceptible to development of transient stuttering they are *not* equally susceptible to persistent stuttering. Clearly large-scale and representative sampling is necessary to determine the precise extent of the sex discrepancy in the incidence of the disorder, but the weight of evidence suggests that the "true" ratio is approximately 3:1.

Among the theorists who have considered the problem of accounting for sex differences in stuttering, West (1958) has probably offered one of the most closely reasoned cases for the "organic" determination of such differences. Briefly, his argument is that male children begin life under the handicap of retarded development which is due to the incompatibility of the endocrine environment under which the male embryo and foetus is nurtured. Damage incurred during gestation and the "struggle for birth" produces anything from "sub-clinical damage" to "obvious chronic pathology"; males suffer more in this way and hence are more prone to retarded development, lowered resistance to disease, a lowered threshold for convulsions (of which stuttering, to West, is an example), and therefore are more susceptible to develop stutters. West concedes that having been thus "weakened" by the character of their early physical environment, the "pressures" exerted by society upon males is bound to exploit and exacerbate the tendencies toward stuttering.

Palmer and Gillett (1938) have suggested that the aetiology of stuttering might profitably be sought in terms of sex-linked meta-bolism. They based this suggestion on the results of an investigation of the pulse rates of normals and stutterers of both sexes. While for nonstutterers the pulse rate of females was faster than that of males, for young stutterers this pattern was reversed. They do not, of course, suggest that variations in pulse rate are directly responsible for stuttering, but argue that such variations, as well as stuttering, have some basis in sex metabolism.

Another study, this time by Ritzman (1943), reported that con-trary to the normal pattern for female subjects to show lower basal metabolic rates than males, female stutterers were higher than males and female controls. Also it was reported that female stutterers showed a tendency toward less marked sinus arrhythmia than did nonstutterers. However, only four female stutterers were available for this experiment, a factor which inspires relatively little confidence in the findings. Andrews and Harris (1964) are of the opinion that the discrepant male/female ratio arises from "inborn constitutional differences", and suggest that two possible genetic explanations might be put forward, that of sex linkage (which they feel is unlikely) or that of sex limitation. They argue that if the mode of transmission were through a single gene the risk of stuttering would be much higher than is actually the case, whether the gene could be assumed to be dominant or recessive. It must, therefore, be assumed that if gene transmission is involved then modifying genes must play an influential role.

In general, the investigations which purport to reflect differences in physical make-up, which would account for the disproportionately high number of males with stutters, are unsatisfactory. Most seem to involve small numbers, poor controls, and dubious logic. How-ever, real differences of this kind cannot be ruled out of consideration especially as there is no compelling evidence that the abnormal sex ratio in stuttering can be accounted for in purely psychological terms.

This alternative psychological account has been expressed by several authors, for example Mills and Streit (1942) express the main argument by protagonists of this view by pointing out that slower development in males is also accompanied by greater pressure to attain fluency. It is supposed that out of this conflict anxiety is produced, and this has the effect of precipitating stutters.

Schuell (1946), in a review of the literature on stuttering in relation to sex differences, points out that the disorder is not only more common among males, but also that the disturbance tends to be more severe in this group. He indicates that the evidence suggests that "physical" causes are at least possible as male infants tend to have more difficult births, are more susceptible to disease, and mature less quickly. However, Schuell argues that the lag in physical, social, and language development of male children leaves them open to unequal competition from female children, and the result must inevitably be frustration, insecurity, and perhaps speech hesitancy. He seems to suggest that the expression of reactions to disadvantageous circumstances could just as well be through some other form of deviant behaviour as through stuttering, for he points out that the sex ratio among delinquents is not unlike that found among stutterers.

In a second publication Schuell (1947) reported upon the results of comparing a small number of boys and girls aged 2–4 years, in terms of disturbances of activities such as eating, sleeping, dressing, etc., for periods from 1 to 6 weeks. The information was derived from interviews with one or both parents of each child. While no statistically significant differences between the sexes in the degree and kind of disturbances manifested were observed, Schuell felt that the data suggested that parents and teachers tend to expect equal performance from children who have not reached the same maturational level. He concluded that the sex differences among stutterers arise out of this combination of physical and psychological factors.

A more incisive study into the psychological factors which might contribute to the differential sex ratio in stuttering was conducted by Bloodstein and Smith (1954). Their inquiry set out to examine the evidence for the proposition that there are higher standards of fluency for boys than for girls, and that such differential expectations contribute to the acquisition of stuttering among males. Tape-recorded samples of speech of young children, aged 4–6 years, were given to 68 "judges" who were required to differentiate the speech samples in terms of the sex of the speaker. The 30 most ambiguous samples were then divided equally and labelled A and B. The samples were then played to groups of college students who were asked to judge whether or not the speaker in the speech sample was a stutterer, one group being told that sample A consisted of boys and sample B of girls, while the other group of judges were given the opposite information.

Two main findings emerged from this study. First, "boys" were not more frequently judged to stutter than were "girls", which suggests that the hypothesis concerning different standards of fluency for the sexes can be rejected. Secondly, it was found that male judges were significantly more prone to make a diagnosis of stuttering than were female judges.

This evidence is, of course, not conclusive for, as Bloodstein and Smith point out, parents may behave in a somewhat different way to independent judges. It may also be said that even if this hypothesis were finally rejected it is still only a limited aspect of the general view that expectations in respect of male children may be higher than is the case for female children. Furthermore, rejection of this hypothesis would not involve simultaneous rejection of the hypothesis advanced by Schuell to the effect that the *same* standards of proficiency are expected of males and females and that the crucial factor is the differential ability to respond with equal ability.

In summary it might be said that there seems little doubt that the incidence of stuttering among males is appreciably higher than that among females by a ratio of approximately 3:1. No satisfactory account, however, has yet been given to account for this finding, both "psychological" and "physiological" theories providing inconclusive evidence. It seems that the solution to this problem may very well provide an invaluable clue to the mechanisms involved in the production of stuttering.

8. *The Relation between Socio-economic Factors and Stuttering*

Little has been done to clarify the relation between socio-economic factors and the occurrence of stuttering, perhaps because such influences appear unlikely to contribute substantially to the explanation of the phenomenon. Most studies carried out in the field fail to control for these factors, and are largely concerned with the availability of subjects. Usually the subjects are drawn from higher socio-economic groups who are more likely to show greater concern and interest in research and treatment of nonfluency.

One of the few detailed studies in this area has been carried out by Morgenstern (1956), who set out to investigate the differential prevalence in stuttering which may occur at different socio-economic levels, and to offer some explanation for any trends which might be observed. Out of some 30,000 children forming the total population of schools surveyed, 350 were judged by speech therapists to be stutterers.

Checking the socio-economic backgrounds of these 350 stutterers against large-scale normative data revealed that the prevalence of the disorder was unrelated to sibling status. However, the prevalence of nonfluency was significantly higher among children of semi-skilled parents and among children of skilled manual workers living in more sparsely populated areas. In addition, stuttering prevalence was lower among the offspring of unskilled parents and where there were crowded housing conditions.

Morgenstern concluded that these results were consistent with Johnson's theory that parental emphasis upon gaining fluency could arouse anxiety which produced stuttering out of normal childhood disfluencies. Such insistence upon rapid achievement of fluent speech would be more likely, it is argued, among parents characterized by socio-economic aspirations.

A more recent study by Andrews and Harris (1964), in which 80 stutterers and 80 nonstutterers were compared, did not reveal any significant relationship between social class and incidence of stuttering, nor was any association observed between the degree and direction of social mobility and stuttering.

On the other hand, an investigation by Douglass and Quarrington (1952) suggests that social mobility may be a factor in some stutterers but not others. Basing their conclusions largely upon case history information and interview, these authors conclude that "interiorized" stuttering (exemplified in inferiority feelings, anti-social behaviour, and anxiety) is associated with social mobility, while those stutterers with overt secondary symptoms (the "exteriorized" type) show no such relationship.

Froeschels (1941) has also argued that socio-cultural influences may influence stuttering, basing this contention upon his experience of both European and American samples. It is claimed that the former tend to avoid the more obvious secondary symptoms (facial contortions, tongue protrusion, etc.) and instead, are more prone to become "Hidden Stutterers" (e.g. avoiding looking into the listener's eyes, and holding a tightly clenched hand in the pocket). Whether or not this observation has validity would require the exercise of careful and painstaking experimental investigation, and the kind of influence proposed here has only the status of an interesting possibility.

It seems unlikely that socio-economic factors are of particular importance to understanding the causes and influences in the field of stuttering, if indeed such factors are relevant at all.

9. *Conclusions*

1. It is commonly assumed that stuttering is a unitary disorder although there is no evidence to this effect and stuttering can take many forms and appear in many different psychological and physical settings.

2. The term "stuttering" covers a large number of different phenomena. Most commonly repetitions, hesitations and blocking of speech, breathing abnormalities, psychological and physical tension, and disturbances of motor activity are found.

3. Figures for the incidence and prevalence of stuttering may show some variation from one culture to another.

4. Prognosis for stuttering is difficult to assess. In general the prognosis for the child stutterer is better than that for the adult.

5. Stuttering, almost invariably, has its onset in childhood. It is not yet clear whether stuttering arises out of "normal" childhood disfluencies.

6. There is no obvious relationship between I.Q. level and stuttering.

7. Stuttering is approximately three times more common among males than females.

8. Stuttering is probably not a significant function of socio-economic factors.

CHAPTER 2

DEFINITION, DIAGNOSIS
AND MEASUREMENT OF STUTTERING

A. DEFINITION

What is stuttering? This may seem a rather obvious question because everyone is sure they can recognize such behaviour when they encounter it. Who is a stutterer? Again, a seemingly superfluous question, as clearly a stutterer is a person who stutters; it is what stutterers do. However, this circular reasoning has been involved in a great deal of stuttering research. The tendency is for investigators to assemble, with no apparent difficulty, a group of people who exhibit certain (usually unspecified) speech disfluencies and to label them "stutterers".

This is not to say that there are insufficient common factors in the speech of certain people to justify grouping them together and thus distinguishing them from other groups. However, it is the case that experimenters rarely define what they mean by "stuttering", and then employ this definition when selecting subjects for their experiments.

When one attempts to define stuttering behaviour, as with so many other "obvious" things, the behaviour becomes less clear-cut, and disagreement among the experts abounds. It is, however, of great importance to be precise when we use the word "stuttering" to describe certain speech behaviour, not only to enable rigorous research to be carried out, but also from the individual's point of view. As Johnson (1956) has so rightly pointed out, there are two occasions when the question of what stuttering *is* becomes of vital importance:

> The first of these is the moment at which the individual, usually when he is a child between two and four years of age, is looked upon for the first time by someone, nearly always his parents, as a stutterer. . . . The other time in the life of an individual when the question becomes crucial is when it becomes . . . "Am I no longer a stutterer?" [p. 202.]

Many attempts have been made to define stuttering behaviour and several of these are referred to in *Stuttering Words*, by Fraser (1963).

A few such definitions will be cited here to give some idea of the kind of attempts which have been made. Johnson (1955) says that "stuttering is an anticipatory, apprehensive, hypertonic avoidance reaction. In other words, stuttering is what a speaker does when (1) he expects stuttering to occur, (2) dreads it, and (3) becomes tense in anticipation of it and in (4) trying to avoid doing it" (p. 217).

Murphy and Fitzsimons (1960) state that

> ... stuttering can be defined as "what a person is". It tells us that self-defensive processes are in action, that anxieties or fears of diffused or specific character are operating, that the person is attempting not only to protect himself but to prove and improve himself also. It reveals to us the level of efficiency with which the person has been able to merge outer reality with inner drives and needs. It is an indicator of the individual's past history; of the problem cores around which his present life is revolving, and around which his future life, in some degree, will be centred. Stuttering gives us an idea of what a person thinks of himself, how he feels about himself, and how he thinks others regard him. Stuttering not only coexists with, but *is a result of*, what a person thinks of himself, feels about himself, and of how he believes others perceive him. [p. 172.]

These definitions tell one something about the person behind the behaviour but give no clue as to how to recognize stuttering behaviour when one encounters it. For this latter purpose a more useful definition is that of Van Riper (1954). For him

> ... the precise definition of stuttering has long presented difficulty. The dictionary refers to it as "hesitating or stumbling in words", but one can hesitate and verbally stumble without stuttering, and one can stutter forcibly without hesitating or stumbling. Most definitions are descriptions, perhaps the best is this; when fixations or repetitions of a sound syllable, or mouth posture are conspicuously unpleasant, most people call it stuttering.

One of the most detailed definitions available is that recently proposed by Wingate (1964). For him the term "stuttering" means:

1. (a) Disruption in the fluency of verbal expression which is (b) characterised by involuntary, audible or silent, repetitions or prolongations in the utterance of short speech elements, namely; sounds, syllables, and words of one syllable. These disruptions (c) usually occur frequently or are marked in character and (d) are not readily controllable.
2. Sometimes the disruptions are (e) accompanied by accessory activities involving the speech apparatus, related or unrelated body structures, or stereotyped speech utterances. These activities give the appearance of being speech-related struggle.
3. Also, there are not infrequently (f) indications or report of the presence of an emotional state, ranging from a general condition of "excitement" or "tension" to more specific emotions of a negative nature such as fear, embarrassment, irritation, or the like. (g) The immediate source of stuttering is some incoordination expressed in the peripheral speech

mechanism; the ultimate cause is presently unknown and may be complex or compound. [p. 488.]

Criticisms of this definition have been offered by Woolf (1965) and replied to by Wingate (1965). One of the points raised by Woolf was that Wingate makes no mention of *avoidance* behaviour. Wingate replied that he deliberately ignored avoidance behaviour since it is an inference and not a fact. This controversy helps to underline the great complexity of the phenomenon for there are some people who are called stutterers who show little speech disturbance although they exhibit all the emotional fears and anticipations that are associated with it; they have become experts in finding synonyms and in performing circumlocutions. This type of stuttering is fairly common and has been described by Freund (1934) as "inneres Stottern" and by Douglass and Quarrington (1952) as "interiorized stuttering". Bloodstein (1960) has gone so far as to say that this avoidance is the most common single feature of a stutterer's speech behaviour. There are, however, few stutterers who are so skilled that they can eliminate all, or nearly all, disfluencies from their speech.

If one accepts Wingate's definition of stuttering behaviour as it stands, then presumably a stutterer is someone whose manner of speaking fits that definition. Unfortunately, it is not too easy to do this because of the qualifications which occur in almost every clause. For example, in "1(c)" one is told that the disruptions "usually occur frequently or are marked in character"; part "3" begins with "Also, there are not infrequently . . .", and "2" begins "sometimes the disruptions are . . .".

One reason for the evident difficulty of speech pathologists in arriving at a rigorous and acceptable definition could be that they are dealing with a phenomenon of multiple causation rather than with a syndrome. One is forced to the conclusion that the majority of investigators regard stuttering as a single disorder, because the general procedure in research is to compare the behaviour of a group of stutterers with the behaviour of a matched group of non-stutterers in some experimental situation. However, more and more frequently the suggestion is being made that stuttering is *not* a single disease entity (e.g. St. Onge and Calvert, 1964), although the only work known to the authors in which research has been specifically designed to study subgroups of stutterers is that of Gray (1966).

One of the factors tending to refute the idea of the single disease entity is the frequent reporting of tremendous variability among stutterers themselves. In some experiments greater variability between *stutterers* has been observed than between stutterers and nonstutterers (e.g. Knott *et al.*, 1959). Such variation has often been the source of negative experimental findings, the difference in response being measured between groups of stutterers and nonstutterers being submerged by the differences *within* the stutterer group. Adding to this evidence and the mass of contradictions and inconsistencies found in research of stuttering, St. Onge (1963) noted that a dictionary definition of "syndrome" showed that this term was hardly applicable to what is known about stuttering. He went on to say that the

> fact that we cannot seem to derive from symptoms a satisfactory syndrome leads us to postulate a multiple etiology. While this sounds nicely academic it is a shallow trick. Not having defined stuttering adequately as a single disorder, by a finely tuned ear for paradox we ascribe it to a variety of causes, but continue to study it as if it were a single disorder. [p. 195.]

Thus, the existence of a "stuttering syndrome" is in some doubt, and the actual definition of what a person does when he is stuttering is fertile ground for argument. It is therefore rather surprising that research workers appear to experience so little difficulty in the selection of their experimental and control groups.

B. DIAGNOSIS

Differential Diagnosis

From the clinician's point of view the diagnosis of stuttering in the adult does not present too much difficulty. The adult usually presents himself to the expert announcing that he stutters and requesting help in its elimination. Whether it is severe or mild it causes him distress and interferes with his day-to-day living. The main differential diagnosis arising here is between stuttering and cluttering, the latter being "characterized by uncontrollable speed which results in truncated, dysrhythmic and incoherent utterance". (*Terminology for Speech Disorders*, 1959.) Sometimes the stuttering may appear to be a symptom of some evident neurosis, psychosis or cerebral injury whose onset is coincident in time with the onset of the basic illness. On the other hand, in the child, the differential diagnosis is usually between stuttering and the normal disfluencies encountered in the speech of nearly all children. Johnson *et al.*, (1956) investigated this in some detail by asking parents what they reacted to when they became worried about their child's speech. Two groups of parents were asked what their children had actually been doing when they were thought to be disfluent or stuttering; one group comprising parents who thought their children were "stutterers" the other including parents who thought their children spoke normally but were "sometimes disfluent".

Table 1 below shows that these two groups of parents were responding to different types of disfluency and indicates where these marked differences occurred.

TABLE 1

Table to show percentages of mothers of "stutterers" (clinical) and mothers of "disfluent" children (control) indicating the type of disfluency their child was exhibiting when he was first thought to be stuttering (or disfluent) (Johnson et al., 1956)

	Clinical mothers	Control mothers
Sound repetition	59	10
Phrase repetition	8	24
Sound prolongation	12	4
Silent intervals	3	41
Interjections	9	21

These data are interesting in showing that the "sometimes disfluent" children had *more* phrase repetitions (I was I was going), *more* pauses and *more* interjections (*uh, er*) than the stuttering children. The mothers of these stuttering children were clearly placing particular emphasis on syllable repetitions (ba-ba-baby) and also to some extent on sound prolongations.

In an analysis of tape-recorded samples of the speech of stuttering and normal speaking children taken about 18 months after the children had been diagnosed as stutterers, Johnson et al. again found similar results. The stuttering children had significantly more syllable repetitions, word repetitions and sound prolongations. The overlap between these samples was quite considerable, 20–30% of the normal speaking children had a greater *total* number of disfluencies than did 20–30% of the stuttering children.

From studies such as these it would appear that the differential diagnosis between "stuttering" and "nonfluency" in the child might be made on the basis of the presence or absence of syllable repetitions and sound prolongations. Williams and Kent (1958) also found that the diagnosis of stuttering was most likely to be made in the presence of syllable repetitions and prolongations, but wonder if the child repeats syllables because his parents think of him as a stutterer or is considered to be a stutterer because he repeats syllables. The main point emerging from these studies is that stuttering and disfluency are not necessarily one and the same thing.

Similar normative data for disfluencies in adults are to be found in Johnson, Darley and Spriestersbach's book, *Diagnostic Methods in Speech Pathology*. These disfluency norms for adults show that the stutterers had many more disfluencies than nonstutterers in both the speaking and reading situations, but again there was considerable overlap. Least overlap between the groups occurred with part-word repetitions (ba-ba-baby). These data are similar to those of Sander (1961) in showing that significantly more disfluencies occur in the speaking than in the reading situation. The significance of this from the point of view of measurement will be discussed in the next section.

Normative data such as those to be found in *Diagnostic Methods in Speech Pathology* are of great importance for the understanding of the phenomenon of stuttering and are, as yet, rare. They are of particular use in the assessment of the speech of a child and for demonstrating to the parents the extent to which the child's disfluencies deviate from the norms of *an American sub-culture*. Similar norms for different cultures are urgently needed so that other relevant comparisons can be made.

Sander (1961) argues that it is also necessary to know the fluency expectations of the listener in a given culture as well as the average number and type of disfluencies actually occurring. Information is also needed concerning the type of disfluency in a given culture which is most likely to elicit the judgement from the listener that the speaker is a stutterer.

Before going on to discuss the reports on diagnosis and evaluation by the listener, it may be useful to illustrate how one writer has attempted to trace the development of stuttering from its first appearance in the young child to its well-established form in the adult. Such an attempt has been made by Bloodstein (1960b), but he has pointed out that his description is of the "average" stutterer's development and that individual stutterers may not go through all four stages or may not even reach the fourth stage.

Bloodstein sees Phase One beginning at pre-school age and continuing until 7 or 8 years of age. During this phase stuttering is episodic; difficulties are experienced on the initial word of a sentence and on conjunctions, prepositions, and pronouns; repetition of syllables is the most striking feature; more stuttering occurs when the child is excited or when he has a lot to say, and the child does not react emotionally to his disfluencies. Apart from these points, Phase One stuttering is similar to that found in adults in that it disappears when any kind of rhythm is imposed on the speech and it shows both the Consistency and the Adaptation effect (see Chapter 6).

Phase Two stuttering shows less fluctuation than Phase One; it occurs primarily when the child gets excited or talks quickly; it occurs primarily on the "major" rather than on "small" parts of speech, and the child now regards himself as a stutterer.

In Phase Three, difficulties with specific situations are found; certain words or sounds are regarded as being especially difficult; there is the use of word substitution; but there is no particular avoidance of speech situations or evidence of fear or embarrassment.

Phase Four is characterized by emotional reactions to speech and sensitivity to the reactions of others, in addition to the other disturbances mentioned above.

Bloodstein hastens to point out that his description of the four phases of development is based on clinical observation only and that the validity of the concept of developmental stages has yet to be shown.

Diagnosis by the Listener

Many theories of stuttering conceive of the listener playing a major role in both the development of the stuttering behaviour and in its persistence.

The majority of experiments in which this role has been investigated have sought to identify what specific types and degrees of speech disfluency are necessary before an individual is labelled by the listener "a stutterer". A few others have sought to determine how the listener really evaluates the stutterer and how he responds to him behaviourally, once having identified him as such.

Most of the research into listener assessments of speech disfluencies has been conducted in the laboratory, with the listener rating the severity of the speech defect from recorded samples, and there is, indeed, some experimental evidence suggesting that this may be a valid procedure. For example, in 1959 Luper showed that judges' ratings of visual, but silent, samples of stuttering shown on film were generally higher than their ratings of the same samples heard on tape. However, Williams *et al.* (1963) argued that in the speaking situation auditory and visual cues are both present when the listener makes his judgements and it is not reasonable to assume that the sound presentation of speech samples will be responded to in the same way as they would be if presented with visual cues as well. To test this they employed three groups of judges to assess frequency and severity of stuttering under conditions of auditory, visual, and audiovisual stimulation, and a *t*-test revealed that the mean number of stutterings under the visual condition was significantly lower than those for the other two groups. These findings suggest that, although visual cues play a part in judged frequency of stuttering (correlation between visual and audiovisual conditions = 0·75), the auditory cues predominate. These results are similar to those of an earlier study by Tuthill (1946) in which the listeners judged there to be the same amount of stuttering whether they had audiovisual or only auditory cues.

The differences between Luper's finding of higher judged frequency of stuttering under visual than auditory conditions, and those of Williams, could perhaps be explained on the grounds that there were more stutterers in Luper's sample who had facial mannerisms. Williams *et al.* comment: "In a few cases, however, the presence of facial distortions influences audio judgements. In these few cases the elimination of visual cues introduces an invalid element in the judgment of severity of incidence of stuttering" (p. 99). As to judgements of severity of stuttering, there was no difference between the visual, auditory, or audiovisual methods, also the reliability judgements of both frequency and severity were higher for auditory and audiovisual cues than for visual cues only.

These experiments have practical as well as academic implications; if the findings are taken at their face value, they suggest that ratings of recorded speech samples will give approximately equivalent results to ratings or scoring made in the face-to-face situation. This in turn means that the stutterer's speech sample can be tape-recorded and replayed several times and so should increase the reliability of scoring as Cullinan *et al.* (1963) suggest. These generalizations should hold good for the majority of stutterers, although there are a few who will be given frequency scores and severity ratings which do not validly represent their actual performance.

Discussing studies on listener reactions, Sander (1965) raises the very important problem concerning the "set" of the listener. This is not relevant when one is attempting to find the most economical way of obtaining reliable judgements of frequency and severity of stuttering to be used in clinical assessment or research, but it may be very relevant to the problem of determining the listener's reactions to speech disfluencies. Sander found that a mother's judgement of the number of stutterings in a 100-word speech sample of a child was affected by prelistening instructions. One set of instructions simply asked the mothers to listen to *what* the child said, the control group being instructed simply to *listen* and the "stuttering" instructions were

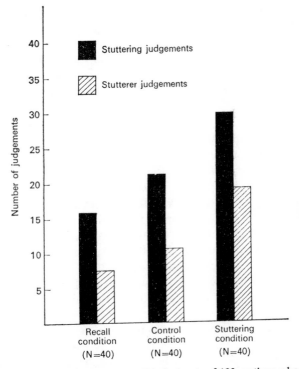

FIG. 2. "Stuttering" and "Stutterer" judgements of 120 mothers who had listened to a child's speech under one of three different prelistening instructions (Sander, 1965).

that the mothers should pay close attention to the *way* the child spoke and to listen for signs of stuttering. Not only were there considerable differences between the groups in the amount they recalled of what the child said, but they also replied differently to the question "did you feel that the child was stuttering?" and "did you feel that the child was a stutterer?". Figure 2 shows the response differences between these three groups.

Williams and Kent (1958) also found differences in response frequency depending upon whether "stuttered interruptions" or "normal interruptions" were asked for first. Whichever instruction was given first produced the most judgements. They commented that their subjects were fairly confused as to what was a "normal" and what was a "stuttered" interruption, the same interruption being quite often marked as both "normal" and "stuttered".

Sander (1965) goes on to point out how rarely investigators have told judges the situational conditions under which the speech samples were obtained and whether the speech sample was considered to be representative of the person's speech behaviour or not. Quite clearly, the speech sample of a child in a high state of excitement would be evaluated very differently by people who know these circumstances compared with those who were told that this was characteristic behaviour.

In another study into the effect of using the word "stuttering" in the instructions, Berlin (1960) provided mothers with the information that this was how the child had generally spoken between the ages of 2 and 5 years of age. He found that all parent groups, except mothers of normal speaking children, "diagnosed more stuttering when the word 'stuttering' was included in the instructions than when it was not" (p. 377). Apart from this there was no difference between the parents of stuttering and nonstuttering children in their evaluations of the children's nonfluencies. These results appear to contradict those of Bloodstein *et al.* (1952), but the latter had simply asked the parents to make the judgement of whether each child stuttered or not with no information on whether this were typical behaviour.

Apart from these difficulties concerning manner of presentation and type of instructions given, the listener clearly reacts to something in the speech samples that evokes from him a judgement of "stuttering". For example, Williams and Kent (1958) found that syllable repetitions and sound prolongations were usually judged as "stuttering", while revisions (I was I was going) were more likely to be regarded as normal disfluencies. Similarly, Young (1961) obtained correlations with severity ratings of 0·83 for part-word repetitions and 0·76 for sound prolongations, where the correlation between severity and revisions was only 0·18. Boehmler (1958) took this one step further by showing that although sound or syllable repetitions were more likely to be called stuttering than any other disfluencies, speech samples containing these types of disfluency were not rated as more severe or extreme. He did find, however, that the more severely the sample was rated the more likely it was to be called "stuttering".

Finally, in Figs. 3 and 4 following, are plotted the relationship between the number of both single-unit and double-unit syllable

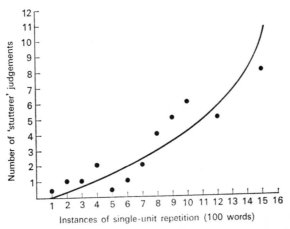

Instances of single-unit repetition (100 words)

FIG. 3. Instances of single-unit repetition (100 words). "Stutterer" judgements of the speaker as a function of frequency of single-unit syllable repetition (120 listeners). The responses of 10 listeners are plotted for each of 12 speech samples containing from 1 to 15 instances of single-unit syllable repetition (Sander, 1963).

repetition and "stutterer" judgements (Sander, 1963). Single-unit syllable repetitions (e.g. Sa-Saturday) evoked only half as many judgements of stuttering as did double-unit syllable repetitions (e.g. Sa-Sa-Saturday), but both types were significantly related to the number of judgements made. The majority of listeners were prepared to make "stutterer" judgements when more than 10 single-unit and 6 double-unit repetitions occurred per 100 words. The different form of the curves reflects the far greater weight given to the double-unit type of repetitions.

It does appear that not only do stutterers produce more part-word or syllable repetitions than do nonstutterers, but that these particular types of disfluency play a significant role in determining the listener's judgements of whether the speaker is or is not a stutterer.

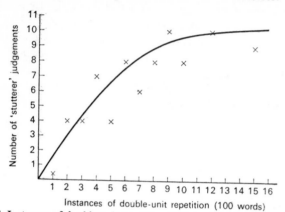

FIG. 4. Instances of double-unit repetition (100 words). "Stutterer" judgements of the speaker as a function of frequency of double-unit syllable repetition (120 listeners). The responses of 10 listeners are plotted for each of 12 speech samples containing from 1 to 15 instances of double-unit syllable repetition (Sander, 1963).

It is perhaps surprising that little has been done to study the effect of number and length of pauses in speech on listener judgements. Both Sander (1961) and Young (1961) advocate the use of rate of speaking as a measure of severity of stuttering, because pauses and hesitations are often an integral part of the speech defect. One of the studies having a bearing on this aspect is that by Wendahl and Cole (1961). These authors investigated whether or not there were any other cues in speech samples, apart from actual disfluencies, which would enable listeners to identify them as having been spoken by stutterers. The sentences used had had all disfluencies deleted from them and had then been carefully matched with those of a nonstutterer so that each listener was presented with several pairs of speech samples about which he had to make his judgement. Not only were the listeners able to discriminate between the speech samples of stutterers and nonstutterers but they judged the stutterers to have a poorer rate of speaking, of speaking with greater force and of using less rhythmical speech. Although the word "stuttering" was used for the stutterer/nonstutterer judgements, this cannot have had any effect on the judgements for rate, force, or rhythm, as different judges were used in each part of the experiment and the word "stuttering" was only used in one part of the experiment. This finding suggests that listeners make their judgement on the basis of more than the actual "moment of stuttering".

In all the studies so far mentioned, the procedure has been to have adults make judgements about the speech of children or adults, but Giolas and Williams (1958) felt that information concerning the reactions of young children to speech difficulties might be of some interest. Accordingly, they designed an experiment in which recordings of three stories were played to children, each story being read with a different speech pattern. The "Interjections Pattern" contained 10% interjections, the "Repetitions Pattern" contained 10% two-syllable and three-syllable repetitions (e.g. b-b-boy and b-b-b-boy) and the third was the "Fluent Pattern". They found that the speech pattern made no difference to the children's enjoyment of the story when they were asked to give their first, second and third choices. However, when asked to give their preference for the story-teller, the 8-year-olds favoured the "Fluent Pattern", gave the "Interjections Pattern" as their second choice and the "Repetitions Pattern" as their third choice. The 5-year-olds placed the speech patterns in the same order, but there was a significant tendency to do so only for the "Fluent" and "Interjections" Patterns. It is interesting that the speech pattern seems not to affect the children's preference for stories when they seem well aware of the sort of speech pattern they like and dislike, but the importance of this study is that it demonstrates that kindergarten children are able to discriminate between fluent and nonfluent speech patterns and have already developed a preference for fluency.

Children and adults both respond to speech disfluencies and evaluate some types more severely than others, but in the studies cited some listeners have been asked to rate the speech as "stuttering" or "not stuttering" while others have asked listeners to rate whether the speaker is "a stutterer" or not. Sander (1963) found that to stutter did not necessarily mean that the person was labelled a stutterer. Sixty-six of 120 mothers reported that a child was stuttering but 30 of these 66 mothers said that they did not think the child was a "stutterer". It seemed to depend largely on what explanation the mother gave for the child's disfluencies whether she called him a stutterer or not. Sander comments that "the type of explanation offered by the listener for the speaker's repetition thus appears to be crucial in shaping the listener's judgement of 'normal' or 'defective' speech" (p. 25). Hence, obviously the more explicit the information about the conditions pertaining at the time the speech sample was recorded, the easier it will be to isolate those factors determining the listener's judgements of "stutterer" and/or "stuttering".

There have been only a few other investigations into the listener's general evaluation of disfluent speech and speakers, and their reactions to these. One is that of Miller and Hewgill (1964), in which they obtained listener's ratings of speech samples differing in number of repetitions or number of vocalized pauses (*uh*). These ratings were on scales representing factors of "Competence", "Trustworthiness" and "Dynamism", and the number of disfluencies, especially repetitions, was found to be related to perceived "Competence" and to a far less extent to "Trustworthiness" and "Dynamism".

Other evidence suggesting that nonstutterers tend to evaluate stutterers in slightly negative or unfavourable terms has been offered by Fransella (1968). In this study the ways in which stutterers and nonstutterers conceptualize people who stutter were compared in terms of a supplied set of concepts. The concepts were rated on the Speech Correction Semantic Differential (Smith, 1962) and the results factor analysed (Fransella, 1965b). It was found that both groups placed the concept "Stutterers" at the "painful", "severe", "difficult" and "tense" pole of the "Pleasantness" dimension and that it tended to be similar in meaning to the concepts "Guilt", "Sensitivity" and "Having a need to belong".

There seems to be some evidence also for the stutterers' observation that listeners will often look away when they begin to speak. Rosenberg and Curtis (1954) observed twenty college students as they talked individually to an experimenter who adopted a "stuttering" or "normal" speech pattern. Their results showed that when listening to the "stutterer" the student maintained significantly less eye contact than with the "normal" speaker. A tendency was also noticed for the student to adapt to the "stuttering" speech and for withdrawal of eye contact to become less marked. This tendency for the listener to adapt to the stutterer's speech was also noted by Ainsworth (1939) who found that the listener's breathing became much less variable as the experiment proceeded. The importance of this listener adaptation in relation to assessing improvement in treatment has been discussed by Trotter and Kools (1955).

There is a great need for further studies into the types of listener response and evaluation with which the stutterer has to contend, and attempts can then be made to relate these to the stutterer's attitudes to the listener. In this way it will be possible to assess the extent to which such attitudes are realistic and hence "normal", and to what extent they are exaggerated and possibly "neurotic".

C. METHODS OF MEASUREMENT

(a) *Severity Rating Scales*

By far the most common way of measuring severity of stuttering, in both the clinical situation and in research, is to rate the speech sample on scales, and Cullinan *et al.* (1963) have made a comparison of the results obtained when several different types of scale were used.

For the basis of their analysis they used 20-second segments of speech which had been selected in another study (Young and Prather, 1962). The 27 samples finally chosen were those that, in the opinion of two speech pathologists, represented the continuum of stuttering severity from very mild to very severe. These 27 speech samples were all rated twice on each of seven scales. Most of the seven types of scale have been used by previous investigators and were as follows.

Equal-appearing intervals with little definition of points:
    I   5-point scale
    II 7-point scale (e.g. Johnson *et al.*, 1963, p. 261)
    III 9-point scale (e.g. Young, 1961; Sherman *et al.*, 1958)
Equal-appearing intervals with points defined in detail:
    IV 7-point scale (e.g. Johnson *et al.*, 1963, pp. 281–2)
Equal-appearing intervals with little definition of points:
    V "likeness to normal speech" (e.g. Williams and Kent, 1958)
    VI "Easiness to listen to"
    VII Direct magnitude-estimation procedure (Prather, 1960)

In this last type of scale judges assign a number or value to a sample of speech which then serves as a standard; values are then assigned to the experimental samples of speech in terms of their severity relative to the standard. Cullinan and his associates thus had 27 samples of speech rated on seven types of scale with each of the seven ratings being made by a different group of undergraduate students ($N = 15$–18).

The results of this study showed that when only one rating was obtained reliability coefficients for one judge ranged from $0·74$ (Scale I) to $0·80$ (Scale III), and the authors concluded that these values were too low "to indicate the use of a single rating from a single judge as an individual predictor". However, reliability coefficients of over $0·90$ could be expected from this single judge if he rated the same speech sample three or more times and took a mean of these ratings. The same pattern of increasing reliabilities can be expected if one takes the mean of a single rating from a number of judges. Thus, for the scales I to VI, four judges rating the same speech sample would be expected to yield a correlation of over $0·90$. The direct magnitude–estimation procedure would be expected to yield somewhat lower correlations, $0·48$ for one judge, $0·79$ for four judges and $0·90$ for ten judges.

Assuming that the reliabilities reported for the single judge doing a number of ratings is representative of a group of judges, then a sufficiently high degree of consistency can be obtained for all types of rating scale, except the direct magnitude–estimation procedure, by either having one judge make three ratings of the same sample or else have four judges make one rating each of the speech sample. Comparisons between each method of rating suggested that there was little difference between them (except for the lower reliability of Scale VII) both in terms of intercorrelations or level of rating.

The authors' conclusions about single ratings from single judges not being reliable enough for individual prediction could perhaps be qualified. In the clinical situation and in research it will be unlikely that the raters will be "incoming undergraduate students". Since the estimated reliability coefficient for these students was over $0·90$ when they did three ratings, it might be predicted that a person with some experience at evaluating and measuring stuttering speech would need to do only two or possibly only one rating to obtain the same level of reliability. This would, of course, have to be demonstrated.

Of particular interest in this study is the fact that six of the seven different types of rating scale were shown to be used in such similar ways. Since the 5-point scale has slightly lower intra- and inter-judge reliabilities than the 7- or 9-point scales, and since scales with equal-appearing intervals and little definition of points are easier to use than the others, it would appear that the 7-point scale of this type has the most to recommend it.

In actual fact the most widely used scale for rating severity of stuttering is probably the Iowa Scale (Johnson *et al.*, 1963) which has the points defined in some detail (p. 281). This tends to make it a rather cumbersome tool for routine clinical use.

Johnson stresses the fact that the scale should only be regarded as a rough measure but that ratings, however crude, ensure some degree of uniformity and comparability of judgements. He also suggests that the clinician should rate more than one speech sample of each stutterer, in addition to having another observer rate the speech samples, so as to increase reliability. Further, he advocates that the stutterer should *rate himself* on the severity of his stuttering periodically throughout treatment. While this latter proposal appears eminently reasonable, self-assessment presents an interesting problem. No great difficulty might be expected to arise if the stutterer used the Iowa Scale, because the 7-points are to some extent objectively defined in terms of percentage of words stuttered and the mean duration of each stutter. However, if the stutterer were to rate himself every month on a 7-point scale without precise definition of points, one must make the basic assumption that the standard against which the stutterer is assessing himself has remained constant. Questioning the stutterer often reveals that this assumption is by no means always reasonable. What often seems to happen is that the degree of stuttering which he now calls "bad" was that which he called "moderate" at the beginning of treatment, and what is now "good" is a level of fluency which was rarely ever experienced in the past. In view of this it seems advisable that, if self-ratings are made on scales with little or no definition of points, the stutterer should be asked to give examples of how he is interpreting the extreme values at the end of each rating session.

In another study concerned with measurement of stuttering Young and Prather (1962) considered that the time and amount of labour needed to rate speech samples of two or three hundred words was "prohibitive", and examined a randomly selected 20-second segment from the total speech sample to see whether this would yield comparable ratings. They also examined whether it made any difference if they always selected the second unit of 20 seconds as opposed to taking a unit at random. While the total speech samples of 50 stutterers had been rated by 40 listeners in a previous study (Young, 1961) the 20-second segments were rated by 14 clinicians on a 9-point scale with little definition of points and no training in rating being given. The correlations indicating the degree of agreement among the raters for each type of speech sample, when the between-listener variance had been removed, were 0·81 for the total speech sample, 0·78 for the randomly-selected sample and 0·74 for the consistently selected sample. The authors attribute the relatively low agreement among the raters to their lack of training and the "exploratory nature of the present study".

TABLE 2

Table to show correlations between ratings of different speech samples (Young and Prather, 1962)

	Randomly-selected sample	Consistently-selected sample
Total sample Randomly-selected sample	0·94	0·82 0·78

On the basis of the figures given in Table 2, the authors suggest that a randomly-selected segment of speech can be regarded as "reasonably representative on average, *for experimental purposes*, of the total samples from which the segments were selected" (p. 258).

In a pilot study to evaluate this method of measurement, and reported in the same paper, the correlation between ratings of the total speech sample and a randomly-selected segment was slightly lower than that previously found (0·88), but this time the number of speech samples was only 15 and the listeners were first-year students instead of the speech clinicians used in the first study.

In view of the possible source of error due to listener variability and segment selection, Young and Prather suggest that "segments be used only when speakers are randomly assigned to treatments or treatment-combinations, or when speakers are given all possible treatment or treatment-combinations" (p. 262).

(b) Analysis of Disfluencies

While there is some indication of lack of agreement in identifying disfluencies, several attempts have been made to define the specific types of disfluency and to measure them.

Johnson *et al.* (1963) advocated the use of eight categories to provide an adequate classification of disfluency types, these being: (i) interjections of sounds, syllables, words or phrases, (ii) part-word repetitions, (iii) word repetitions, (iv) phrase repetitions, (v) revisions, (vi) incomplete phrases, (vii) broken words and (viii) prolonged sounds. In addition to describing standard methods for obtaining and analysing speech samples, Johnson *et al.* include norms for reading rates and frequency of the different types of disfluency for both adults and children, stutterers and nonstutterers, in the United States of America.

TABLE 3

Table to show means, ranges and standard deviations of measures of disfluency and rate based on 200 words spoken by 50 adult males with the problem of stuttering (Young, 1961)

Disfluency category	Mean number of disfluencies	Percentage of total disfluencies	Range of no. of disfluencies	S.D.
Interjections	19·2	36·7	2–95	16·8
Part-word repetitions	14·4	27·5	0–79	16·1
Word-phrase repetitions	5·5	10·6	0–28	5·1
Prolongations	10·5	20·0	0·70	15·5
Revisions	2·7	5·1	0–8	1·8
Total[1]	52·3	100·0	4–223	40·8
Time	*Mean number of seconds* 134·0	*Range of No. seconds* 61–595		

[1] Sum of measures for all disfluency categories.

Modifications of the disfluency categories have been suggested by both Young (1961) and Sander (1961). Young reduced the eight categories to five by combining word and phrase repetitions, by extending prolonged sounds to include broken words, and revisions to include incomplete phrases. In addition to this modification he measured time taken to speak, since he felt that the pauses in speech so characteristic of the stutterer might well be taken account of when the listener was rating severity. The means, standard deviations and ranges obtained by Young for the five types of disfluency and rate of speaking are given below in Table 3.

Young intercorrelated all these different disfluency categories, time, and total disfluencies, and the resulting matrix can be seen in Table 4.

TABLE 4

Table to show intercorrelation matrix for dependent variable and independent variables 1 through 6[1] (Young, 1961)

	1	2	3	4	5	6	T^2
0	0·68[3]	0·45	0·83	0·37	0·76	0·18	0·85
1		0·76	0·52	0·26	0·55	0·06	0·76
2			0·33	0·42	0·33	0·13	
3				0·39	0·65	0·16	
4					0·15	0·29	
5						0·02	

[1]0: rated severity of stuttering;   1: speaking time;   2: interjections;
    3: part-word repetitions;   4: word-phrase repetitions;
    5: prolongations;   6: revisions.
[2] Sum of disfluency categories 2 through 6 (total number of disfluencies).
[3] For df = 48 rs of 0·279 (5 %) and 0·361 (1 %) are significantly different from zero.

In a second part of his experiment, Young demonstrated that the regression equation based on 100 samples of speech could not be used for predicting an individual's ratings of severity from time taken to speak and frequency of "repetitions", because the assumptions of linearity and homoscedasticity were not satisfied. The category of "repetitions", he suggests, could be used as an operational definition of disfluency, this being "the number of words in relation to which a part-word repetition, a sound prolongation, a broken utterance, or unusual stress was observed" (pp. 42–3).

Another way of defining disfluent words has been suggested by Sander (1961). In his study he considered a word "disfluent" if it involved "prolonged sounds, was classified as a broken word, was involved in a sound, syllable, or word repetition, or was interrupted by an interjection. Words preceded by interjections or involved in phrase repetitions were not counted as disfluent words" (p. 24). Sander's "disfluent" words are clearly very similar to Young's "repetitions". However, Sander's main aim was to assess the relia-bility of the Iowa Speech Disfluency Test. This test involves the stutterer or nonstutterer reading a standard passage of prose and speaking spontaneously for about 3 minutes. Sander had a group of 34 stutterers repeat this test after a 24-hour interval, using the same passage of prose to read but a different speaking task. Measures were the number of disfluencies in each of the test's eight categories, the number of "disfluent words", and the rate of utterance.

Since total disfluencies and "disfluent words" correlated 0·87 for speaking and 0·86 for reading, Sander concluded that these were high enough for a simple count of "disfluent words" to be used as a measure of disfluency. This he suggested should be combined with a measurement of rate of utterance, since there was a correlation of 0·86 between this and number of disfluencies for reading, and 0·81 for speaking. Reading rate and speaking rate correlated 0·90.

Much lower correlations were obtained between the disfluency measures for the reading and speaking tasks, being 0·72 for total disfluencies and 0·70 for "disfluent words". These values are in line with Johnson et al.'s reported correlations of 0·67 and 0·75 between oral reading and two types of speaking task for a group of stutterers. Particularly interesting is Johnson's finding that when similar calculations were carried out on the disfluencies of *nonstutterers* on reading and two speaking tasks, the resulting correlations were only 0·13 and 0·45. Other differences between the speech characteristics of stutterers and nonstutterers will be discussed later. It is important to note that Sander's obtained distributions of disfluency scores for speaking and oral reading are markedly skewed, and that the range of scores is large (see Table 5).

TABLE 5

Table to show means, standard deviations, and ranges of total disfluencies, disfluent words, and time for Sessions I and II of the Reading and Speaking Tasks (N = 40)
(Sander, 1961)

	Speaking			Reading		
	Mean	S.D.	Range	Mean	S.D.	Range
Total Disfluencies:						
Session I	78·1	55·4	8–230	48·2	64·3	0–270
Session II	81·2	56·6	15–255	46·0	54·7	1–210
Disfluent Words:						
Session I	38·2	33·4	1–134	29·0	38·7	0–184
Session II	40·0	32·0	3–122	29·1	35·4	0–160
Time in Seconds:						
Session I	242·4	207·3	86–1235	218·4	206·9	89–1028
Session II	237·7	167·4	92–853	198·7	141·0	85–782

He used the Pearson product–moment correlation to calculate the degree of relationships between the number of disfluencies on the first test occasion and the second 24 hours later. This statistic assumes that the scores are from a bivariate normal distribution which is clearly not the case in Sander's data, but the test–retest correlations he reports of from $0 \cdot 91$ to $0 \cdot 97$ are so high that there is obviously a strong relationship. Two other things indicate that there was considerable stability in the disfluencies of this group of stutterers: (a) inspection of Table 5 shows there to be very little variation in the means and standard deviations of the disfluency scores; and (b) Sander compared each stutterer's disfluencies with the disfluency norms reported by Johnson et al. (1963) (Tables 37–39, pp. 222–4) and placed each in the corresponding decile group. On retest about half the stutterers maintained their original decile positions for both the speaking and reading tasks, and about a third shifted only one decile.

Sander's finding that changes in the number of disfluencies in one task are not necessarily accompanied by changes on the other task underlines the importance of using both speaking and reading tasks when attempting to assess change in stuttering frequency over time. The fact that Sander demonstrated considerable consistency in disfluency scores and rate of utterance over a 24-hour period must not blind one to the fact that in clinical situations assessment of change is likely to be in terms of weeks rather than hours. A more rigorous test of reliability of a scale might be to measure disfluencies, say, once each month, in those stutterers not receiving treatment.

It is a common observation that one of the most characteristic features of stuttering is its day-to-day variability. Milisen (1957) goes so far as to conclude that the quantification of the stutterer's speech behaviour "need not involve highly accurate measurements of overt symptoms or attitudes, because the conditions change so markedly from one period to another and from one situation to another". In spite of this the aim of the research worker will always be to measure the phenomenon he is investigating as accurately as possible, and until more is known about the causes of these fluctuations and what makes one day "good" and other "bad" from the stutterer's point of view, serial testing in any research project dealing with treatment must assume that these fluctuations are random with respect to time of day, day of week and month of year.

D. RATE OF READING AND SPEAKING

Enough has been said about rate of utterance in the preceding section on measurement to justify a short account of studies which have directly or indirectly investigated the rate at which stutterers speak. For example, it was mentioned that Young measured reading rate and found that this correlated with severity rating 0·68, and with interjections 0·76, and Sander (1961) reported that reading rate correlated with speaking rate 0·90.

In an earlier study Bloodstein (1944) measured reading rate in two ways, (i) he divided the total number of words by the total time taken to read, and (ii) he derived a measure of nonstuttering reading rate by eliminating the time taken over stuttered words. He then correlated these measures with frequency of stuttering and found it to be −0·88 for overall reading rate and −0·77 for nonstuttering reading rate. His group of stutterers showed a slower nonstuttering reading rate than a group of normal speakers. Likewise, in a study designed to see whether there was anything in nonstuttered speech that would differentiate stutterers from nonstutterers, Wendahl and Cole (1961) found that judges rated the stutterers "nonstuttering speech" as being slower than that of normally fluent persons.

Several factors may contribute to this general slowing down of the stutterer's rate of reading (most studies have been concerned with reading rather than speaking rate). They may hold on to a syllable or pause unduly before a difficult syllable (Robbins, 1935), they may alter their breathing rhythm (Van Riper, 1936), or there may be an inhibitory or "heel-dragging" quality to their speech.

Cullinan (1963) also used a total or overall reading time measure and a nonstuttered reading rate in syllables per minute. He decided on this unit of measurement because more stuttering occurs on polysyllabic words than on monosyllabic words so that the non-stutterer's reading rate might be greater than the overall reading rate because the nonstuttered words would tend to be shorter. The mean overall reading rate and the mean nonstuttered reading rate for each of five readings on each of 3 days are plotted in Figs. 5 and 6. The means for overall reading rate in syllables per minute are all below those previously reported by Darley (1940), as indeed were those of Bloodstein (1944). In both figures it can be seen that there is an increase in reading rate from reading to reading, but Cullinan found that an individual's performance from day to day was too unreliable for overall or nonstuttering reading rate to be used as an index of stuttering behaviour.

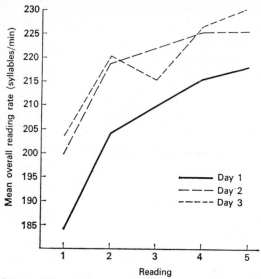

FIG. 5. **Mean** overall reading rate for each of five readings of the 300-word passage by 23 stutterers on each of 3 days (Cullinan, 1963).

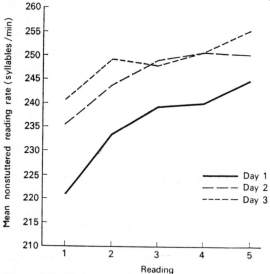

FIG. 6. Mean nonstuttered reading rate for each of the five readings of the 300-word passage by 23 stutterers on each of 3 days (Cullinan, 1963).

There is thus some evidence that the reading rate of stutterers is slower than that for nonstutterers even when one has made allowance for time spent in actual stuttering behaviour; that listeners respond to this slowness is also suggested by the finding of Wendahl and Cole (1961), and the overall slowness is reflected in the correlation between severity rating and time taken to read of 0·68 reported by Young.

It has been suggested that this reading slowness is also to be found in the silent reading rate of stutterers (Murray, 1932). In a recent study (Fransella and Beech, 1965) a mean silent rate of reading a list of words was reported as being 42·44 seconds for stutterers and 36·1 seconds for nonstutterers, but this slightly slower silent reading rate for stutterers did not differ significantly from that of the nonstutterers on a Mann–Witney U-test. The apparent contradictory results of these studies are probably attributable to the method of analysis used. Statistical methods have changed considerably since 1932 and it may be that the finding of Murray, that stutterers were two grades below the control group in silent reading rate, would also not be significant on a statistical test in view of the very wide range of scores on such tests. However, it is interesting that the trends observed in these studies are in the same general direction.

Conclusions

1. No adequate definition of stuttering has yet been suggested. One of the more detailed operational definitions is that of Wingate (1964), but this has certain limitations.

2. Evidence is steadily accruing, suggesting that stuttering cannot be described as a syndrome.

3. Stuttering and disfluency are not necessarily the same thing.

4. Speech is likely to be judged "stuttering" if it contains syllable repetitions and sound prolongations.

5. The listener is still able to detect abnormalities in samples of speech from which all disfluencies have been deleted.

6. The 5-year-old child already seems to have a preference for speech patterns.

7. The stutterer may tend to be evaluated in unfavourable terms by both stutterers and nonstutterers.

8. Where ratings of severity of stuttering are concerned, the evidence suggests that a 7-point scale with little definition of points

may be useful. To obtain a high level of reliability, each rating should be made at least twice or else more than one judge should rate each speech sample.

9. The rating of a randomly-selected 20-second segment of speech from a total speech sample may be sufficiently representative of the total speech sample to be useful for experimental purposes.

10. Simplified methods of quantifying disfluencies, as suggested by Sander and Young, correlate well with ratings of severity, as does speed of utterance.

11. Measures should be taken in both the reading and speaking situations as the correlations between them tend to be low.

12. Stutterers tend to read more slowly than nonstutterers even when time taken in stuttering has been taken into account.

CHAPTER 3

THEORIES OF STUTTERING

1. *Introduction*

The activity of explaining is a familiar experience in everyday life and, as often as not in the context of daily experiences, we attempt to explain some new happening or event in terms of an existing framework of knowledge. Frequently we find that there is a reluctance to abandon an old and previously satisfactory explanation, and new accounts or theories concerning the interrelationships between things or events have to be forced upon us by significant increases in our store of information. Radical changes as a result of increased information are, perhaps, most familiar in the physical sciences, the progression from Ptolemy's view of the earth as a fixed body in the centre of the universe to later views expressed by Copernicus, Kepler, Newton and Einstein being an example of this.

Stuttering theory, in general, does not reflect the kind of progressive change and refinement which one might have expected from a developing science. To some extent the field may suffer as a result of being treated as one of the social sciences, and perhaps it is the case that the "hard facts" which are necessary to the foundation of a satisfactory science are lacking and difficult to discover. Whatever the roots of the problem may appear to be it is certainly the case that no very satisfactory theory of stuttering has yet been formulated. However, to some extent the formulation of explanations may have operated as a stimulus to experiment, and the field of stuttering is now characterized by the growth of basic experimentation and sound methodological considerations.

The principal guide to theory construction should be that of accounting for, or describing, the functional relations between as many of the available facts as possible. It is also usual to insist upon prediction and control rather than upon "understanding" in formulating theoretical accounts. To some extent it might be that one is forced to put forward an explanation which emphasizes "understanding"; for example, in the case of earthquakes and similar natural phenomena prediction and control may be difficult or impossible to achieve. Theories of stuttering have been generally characterized by an emphasis upon one or several of the available facts, rather than attempts to encompass and relate all information, but, on the other hand, it is also the case that most theories have, quite properly, concentrated attention upon prediction and control of the stuttering disorder, rather than upon simply "understanding". The second of these two aspects of theoretical orientation seems to be the natural outcome of "pressure to treat" as well as the obvious availability of external controls which modify the abnormality in some way.

When one is considering the nature of the theory itself, clearly one has two expectations in mind, the first of which is concerned with empirical observations. Without a broad basis in statements of fact a theory is less likely to be of value. In the field of stuttering the important facts are generally reproducible and deal with a satisfactory proportion of the variance in the observed behaviour, for example the tendency for less stuttering to occur on successive occasions of reading the same passage. In other cases the nature and quality of the facts brought forward as the basis of, or in support of, a particular theory seem to have a less solid foundation, for example neurological abnormalities.

The theories can indeed be differentiated both in terms of the number of facts which are dealt with, the quality and character of these facts, and the order of importance of these facts for the theory. However, it can reasonably be argued that empirical observations, systematically gathered under controlled conditions, are available in sufficient (though small) number to warrant the formulation of theories.

The second prerequisite is concerned with the kind of hypothetical and theoretical propositions involved. It is sufficient to regard theoretical propositions as the more general formal statements, while hypotheses are concerned with more specific propositions. The important considerations here are those of the extent to which hypothesis and theory are tied to observable facts and evidence, and the degree to which the general formulations permit the deduction of new facts or evidence as yet unobserved.

Broadly speaking there are two main kinds of theory available in accounts of stuttering, the Reductive and the Constructive. The former is concerned with the accounts in which the variables employed in explanation are drawn from observations of the kind assigned to neurophysiological level of description. West's theory is an example of this type. In the Constructive theory the phenomena under consideration are dealt with in terms of more abstract constructs, and Sheehan's model clearly falls into this category.

Both types of theory can, of course, be useful, and both have advantages and disadvantages. In the case of the two theories mentioned above, for example, West's theory avoids the complications which attend the use of hypothetical constructs, but runs into the difficulty of demonstrating malfunctioning of neurological processes. On the other hand, Sheehan is able to capitalize upon a wealth of existing data concerning conflict situations in building his theory, but meets greater difficulties in extrapolating from it.

The following section is concerned with a brief survey of some of the important theories in the field of stuttering. In selecting the six theories for presentation an attempt has been made to provide a reasonable cross-section of the views expressed, although the emphasis has been upon those with experimental and research data forming an integral part of their construction or testing. This last-named consideration has, for example, led to the exclusion of the psychoanalytic theory of stuttering. As has been pointed out earlier, none of the theories could be described as entirely satisfactory, and none can stand up to detailed and searching criticism. Nevertheless, their value lies, at least in part, upon the impetus which they give to research, and also in the added emphasis they bring to special and particular aspects of the field.

2. *Stuttering as a Perceptual Defect: Cherry and Sayers*

The method by which serious disruptions of normal fluency can be produced was first reported by Lee (1950). This method, called delayed-playback speech, is one in which the speaker's utterances are fed back to him with a short delay of approximately $\frac{1}{5}-\frac{1}{10}$ second. The speech disturbance produced in this way suggests that normal fluency depends, to some extent, upon the efficiency of a "feedback" system by which the speaker monitors his speech.

Without making claims to a formal theory of stuttering, Cherry and Sayers (1956) set out to examine the proposition that stuttering could be considered to be a perceptual defect. The suggestion is that stuttering is the result of an instability of the feedback loop, and their experiments have been aimed at breaking the closed-cycle feedback action and examining the effects upon the nonfluency of stutterers.

The starting point adopted by Cherry and Sayers is that of shadowing, this being used as a means of interfering with the monitoring process, by which the attention of one speaker is transferred from the sound of his own voice to that of another speaker. Shadowing, simultaneous speaking by the stutterer and a person with normal fluency, and other similar experiments were found to produce "near normal" speech among stutterers, and Cherry and Sayers suggest that continued exercises along these lines might change the perceptual habits of the stutterer.

However, in these experiments the speech of the stutterer is subject to the external control of attention, while under normal conditions speech is subject to the control of feedback processes both through air-conduction and bone-conduction pathways. It is important to ask whether both pathways exert a similar influence upon the perceptual habits which produce stuttering.

Air-conducted sound was eliminated by blocking the ears, but had no consistent effect; on the other hand, a loud masking tone, eliminating air *and* bone conduction, produced a striking increase in the fluency of stutterers. Further experimentation suggested that blocking of very low frequency tones in the speaker's voice was necessary for efficient control of the stutter, and Cherry and Sayers point out that whispering produced similarly effective results. All this suggested that the low frequency tones, monitored through bone-conduction pathways, are responsible for the perceptual abnormality associated with stuttering, although Cherry and Sayers do not, of course, claim that this abnormality is the necessary *cause* of stuttering.

Three main alternatives to account for the results were considered. First, the authors say, it could be that their findings simply illustrate the operation of a distraction which serves to inhibit stuttering. Secondly, it could be argued that the loud masking tone presents a new and unusual situation to the stutterer, although this seems to be an unlikely explanation as little or no change occurs with repeated application of the procedure. Thirdly, as the masking noise was extremely loud, this encouraged stutterers to speak loudly and this factor might alone have accounted for the improvement. This was easily checked by asking subjects to speak quietly during the operation of the masking tone, and the results eliminated the "loud speaking" explanation.

It would be possible to account for several other well-documented phenomena of stuttering in terms of the Cherry and Sayers hypothesis, for example the rhythm effect might be another means of interfering with feedback processes through altered attention, and the adaptation effect might be interpreted as a reflection of a pro- gressively reduced necessity to "monitor" one's speech productions. However, the crucial issue raised in connection with the Cherry and Sayers hypothesis is that of whether the effects of delayed auditory feedback resemble stuttering.

The most important contribution in this respect comes from Neelley (1961) who concluded that there was little evidence for any similarity between nonfluencies produced by stuttering and those resulting from delayed auditory feedback (D.A.F.). This conclusion is based upon three main sources of evidence:

1. That there is little evidence for the adaptation effect in D.A.F. while this effect is consistently found in stuttering research.
2. The listener can distinguish without difficulty between stuttering and D.A.F.-induced nonfluencies from tape recordings.
3. That listeners were unable to differentiate stutterers from non-stutterers in terms of their responses to D.A.F. conditions. This point, taken in conjunction with the preceding one, suggests that delayed auditory feedback produces a type of nonfluency which is different from stuttering.

These points are serious but probably not fatal to the hypothesis that stuttering and D.A.F. effects are related. One could argue, for example, that too little time has been spent upon D.A.F. tasks to allow adaptation to appear, and that one should not be too disturbed to find that the speech difficulties produced by D.A.F. differ from stuttering, as the latter has usually been the result of prolonged modification and change of the original nonfluency.

A more detailed account of D.A.F. research is presented in Chapter 7 but, so far as the theory of a defect in monitoring among stutterers is concerned, it can be said that we have here a genuine and interesting alternative approach to the problems of the stutterer. Further extension and development of the D.A.F. hypothesis would undoubtedly be of considerable general as well as specific value.

3. *Organic Theory of Stuttering: West*

In his formal statement of his views concerning stuttering West (1958) makes it quite clear that he is an "agnostic" in the sense that he feels that the available facts do not allow us to be sure about the basic aetiology of stuttering. Nevertheless, he is prepared to "speculate" about one possible organic cause of stuttering because, in his opinion, such an explanation is more in accord with the available evidence than the alternative views which have been expressed.

He begins by setting out the kind of facts which he believes should be dealt with by any theory of stuttering. These are, that it is predominantly a phenomenon which appears in childhood; is more prevalent among males; is associated with cerebral dominance; has familial characteristics; is associated with multiple births and late development of speech; is insidious in onset; is convulsive (i.e. involves muscular spasms); and is related to situations where the stutterer feels that the abnormality is likely to occur.

He does not rule out the possibility that psychological factors play some part in the disturbance, but takes the view that one can frequently demonstrate psychological "triggers" of organic disturbances and that one should not be surprised to find that this is true for stuttering. Indeed, the susceptibility of stuttering to psychological factors lends weight to his argument that stuttering is a kind of convulsive disorder, related to the epilepsies. Both epilepsy and stuttering are convulsive; both are more common among males; both are susceptible to states of heightened emotionality and occur more frequently in childhood; both have a familial element; and both are "reflexive" in that fear of an attack can precipitate the disorder.

West is clearly aware that it is necessary to do more than provide evidence for a superficial resemblance between epilepsy and stuttering. He attempts to establish this more direct relationship by pointing out that Kopp (1934) reports that stutterers, as a group, are characterized by raised blood sugar ratings. This, he suggests, might reflect the failing attempt on the part of the organism to prevent the occurrence of convulsions, and but for the operation of this compensatory mechanism the convulsions might be more severe (see Chapter 4).

In essence he argues that there is a reasonable case for regarding stuttering as a partially compensated pyknolepsy, i.e. a form of epilepsy characterized by many minor convulsions which, being confined to the musculature involved in speech, leads to brief but frequent arrest of vocalization.

The great difficulty with West's theory is not so much that it runs counter to existing evidence but that there is no direct and positive evidence to support it. It is true that Berry's (1932) report suggests that stuttering sometimes is found as one of the sequelae of encephalitis and epilepsy, and it is possible that these disorders produce structural changes which are like those which might be found among stutterers. Travis and Knott (1937) have also reported disturbances in the electrical activity of the brain associated with stuttering, a finding which would support any "organic" theory. However, neither Moravek and Langova (1962) nor Rheinberger et al. (1943) were able to confirm this finding in their studies.

Nevertheless, some researchers still report differences in the electrical activity of the brain between stutterers and controls (e.g. Douglass, 1943; Knott et al., 1959). But perhaps one of the most recent and compelling studies is that reported by Jones (1966), who based his study upon suggestions made by Travis (1931) and Bryngelson (1935) which, taken together, suggest that stutterers might be characterized by an imperfect degree of cerebral dominance and/or bilateral cerebral activity.

Jones, basing his assumption upon the work of Penfield and Roberts (1959), argues that most people use one or other cerebral hemisphere for speech. However, Branch et al. (1964) have reported that some individuals are characterized by mixed cerebral dominance which might be demonstrable in several modalities. If stutterers were found to have mixed dominance, then it would be of interest to examine the effects of an attempt to transfer the influence to one or other hemisphere, and Jones was fortunate to find four individuals with one-sided cerebral lesions in the region of speech areas, on whom to test this effect.

Using Wada's intracarotid amytal test and other measures confirmed that there seemed to be bilateral representation of the speech mechanism in these four stutterers. Most striking, however, were the results of a one-sided operation for the lesions unrelated to the onset of the stutter; completely normal speech was restored to all patients and no relapse was noted even after 3 years of follow-up in one case. The final significant finding in this study was that use of the intracarotid amytal test after operation suggested that speech dominance was no longer bilateral and that transfer of influence to one hemisphere only had been accomplished.

4. *Perseverative Theory of Stuttering: Eisenson*

This is not so thoroughgoing an "organic" theory as West's, but it does assume a strong constitutional element is present in stuttering. The central proposition in Eisenson's theory (1958) states that the constitutional factor, which differentiates stutterers from nonstutterers, is a predisposition to perseverate, i.e. the former group are susceptible to the persistence of mental or motor activities, after the removal of the stimulus to such activities, for a longer period of time than are nonstutterers. In this sense stuttering is regarded as an example of a perseverative activity.

Such a theory needs to establish two important facts; first, that an exaggerated tendency to perseverate is a general characteristic of stutterers which can be demonstrated on a number of different tasks and modalities, and secondly, that there is a direct relationship between perseverative behaviour in general, and stuttering.

Eisenson is apparently aware of the difficulty of demonstrating a general trait of perseveration among normal speakers, but has carried out experiments of his own to test this important proposition in respect of stutterers. In one such experiment he reports finding that stutterers experience greater difficulty in shifting or varying an existing "set" than is the case for nonstutterers. He also quoted Falck (1955) as showing that the tendency to exhibit tonic blocks is associated with perseveration as a personality trait.

Eisenson refers to King's study (1953) as providing yet more direct evidence for his theory although it is important to note that King, like most researchers in this field, could find no evidence for the existence of a general trait of perseveration. However, King's data suggested that stutterers experienced greater difficulty than nonstutterers in effecting rapid changes in response set, although this difference was not clear-cut and the two groups showed much overlap. In other words, while the two groups differed on average on the tasks, some stutterers behaved like nonstutterers and some nonstutterers appeared as perseverative.

Eisenson goes on to develop his theory by considering some of the factors which appear to be related to increments and decrements in the amount of stuttering. Such factors he seems to consider are often related to the kind of words which carry the burden of meaning in speech (e.g. nouns, verbs, long words, first words), and it is these words which are more frequently stuttered.

He argues that difficulty in reading aloud, for example, varies directly with the meaningfulness or *propositionality* of the text, and that if we attempt to reduce the propositionality by talking nonsense, or talking to children, or from memory, then speech difficulty is also reduced.

As an example of the influence of propositionality Eisenson examines the adaptation effect. He recognizes that it is possible to account for the usual progressive development of fluency with repeated readings of the same passage in terms of lowered anxiety, and says that other variables may also play a part in producing the adaptation effect. However, Eisenson argues that re-reading will involve changes in propositionality, and this may, at least in part, account for increasing fluency. He points out that changes in the pattern of speech can be observed with re-reading, such as slurring, increased rate, greater dependence upon memory, and changes in stress and sounds, so that it cannot be argued that we are dealing with repetitions of precisely the same situation; real changes may be occurring in the meaning of the material which could alone be responsible for the so-called adaptation phenomenon (see Chapter 6).

In essence, therefore, Eisenson is postulating a transient disruption of propositional speech as the basis for degree of stuttering.

According to his theory not all stutterers are constitutionally inclined to perseverate; approximately 60% are so, but the remaining number are simply individuals for whom the external factors which promote perseveration (increased propositionality, situational difficulties, etc.) have combined to produce a stutter. The latter group are not, therefore, regarded as having some defect in neurological make-up.

But do all constitutional perseverators necessarily become stutterers? This depends, according to Eisenson, upon whether the environment affords opportunities for certain aspects of environmental circumstances to become associated with speech. He points out that repetitive speech is common in early childhood, but believes that some individuals struggle against the predisposition to perseverate. In the course of this struggle for fluency all kinds of contortions are produced and the word is finally spoken in spite of these rather than because of them. In time, it is argued, the stutterer comes to regard the struggle as necessary to release the block, so that both learning as well as constitution play an important part in the development of the stutter in this theory.

The 40% of stutterers regarded by Eisenson as "non-organic" are said to have the same difficulty as the "organics" with propositional speech, but in these individuals the mechanisms contributing to the difficulty are different. For the "non-organics" it is assumed that conflict exists between the desire to speak and the desire to remain silent, and perseveration (stuttering) occurs when the approach to speech is blocked in some way, for example by heightened anxiety. Such a situation might, according to Eisenson, lead to greater difficulty with non-propositional speech in this group, as the conflict might generalize to situations not previously experienced as "difficult".

In essence the central difference between the "organic" and "non-organic" stutterer is that on the one hand there is a disturbance of linguistic formulation, while on the other there is an anticipatory avoidance reaction to speaking.

According to Eisenson several factors may play a part in predisposing the "non-organic" individual to develop stutters and continue to manifest speech defects long after the period during which these defects can be considered to be "normal". One of these factors, he suggests, is a disposition toward a generalized antagonism between needs, while another is a tendency toward greater generalization of experiences. A third factor may be an inclination to inhibit the expression of personal thoughts and feelings to a greater degree than is usual, and Eisenson states that the environment of stutterers belonging to this group may also be implicated, especially if this environment is harsh, restrictive and too demanding.

Two things are immediately obvious in evaluating this theory; first, that the evidence on which it is based is relatively weak, and secondly, that the theory is compounded of many elements without the relation between these elements being very clearly formulated. In a sense Eisenson admits a further weakness in his theory when he states that most of the factors he has associated with stuttering can be found among children who acquire normal fluency, and it is clear that this model lacks the kind of rigour which is ordinarily required in a theoretical formulation.

This is not to say that certain central aspects of the theory are unamenable to experimental test as it is a relatively simple matter to examine quite directly both the notion concerning perseveration and that concerning propositionality difficulty. Martin (1962) has in fact tested the perseveration hypothesis in two ways, first by comparing stutterers and nonstutterers in terms of their performance on tests of perseveration (although intercorrelations between such tests are too low to be confident that one is measuring the same things), and secondly by testing the deduction from Eisenson's theory that the degree of perseveration as measured should be related to the amount of stuttering observed. Employing 52 stutterers and 109 nonstutterers, between the ages of 8 and 13, in his study Martin was unable to confirm either part of the perseveration hypothesis.

Weakness of the evidence upon which the theory is based, together with negative findings and a general lack of precision in its formulation, makes this one of the less attractive theories of stuttering.

5. *An Expectancy Theory of Stuttering: Wischner*

This theory represents an interesting departure from the more global approach adopted by several other theorists in that Wischner (1948, 1950, 1952) concentrates his attention upon one of the outstanding observations concerning modification of stuttering—the so-called "anticipation effect". The kind of evidence which he considers might be summarized as follows:

1. Several investigations have indicated (e.g. Knott *et al.*, 1937) that the stutterer can accurately predict in excess of 90% of words with which he will experience difficulty.

2. Johnson and Solomon (1937) report that the anticipations of stuttering difficulty are largely correct even when such predictions have been made several days prior to the assessment. This, of course, reduces the possibility that the subject is unduly influenced by specific decisions made.

3. It has been shown (Johnson and Sinn, 1937) that elimination of words for which there is stuttering expectancy reduces the degree of stuttering produced to an insignificant level.

4. It has been reported that there appears to be some consistency in the judgement of stutterers respecting those specific words for which they anticipate difficulty (Johnson and Ainsworth, 1938).

5. Milisen (1938) has pointed out that his experience suggests that only rarely do stutterers experience difficulty with words which

have been anticipated as "not difficult", and only rarely does he *not* stutter on words which are anticipated as "difficult".

6. Finally, Van Riper and Milisen (1938) have reported that stutterers are able to correctly predict the degree of difficulty they are likely to experience for particular words in terms of whether the stutter will be of short, medium, or long duration.

As Wischner points out, it is possible to argue that one mechanism involved in "expectancy" is that concerning preparatory set. The argument would be that preliminary inspection of words in a text, for example, would reveal certain cues associated with particular words and, should these cues be unfavourable, there may be rehearsal movements which would provide a "set to stutter".

It would also be argued that these "cues" which are detected by the stutterer are related to the amount of anxiety they evoke. Van Riper, for example, has subdivided such cues into those concerned with generalized stuttering expectancy and those concerned with specific stuttering expectancy. The former have to do with the similarity of the situations or contexts in which speech is to occur, while the latter are concerned with those specific words with which the subject has previously experienced difficulty.

Wischner states that there is evidence for both specific and general expectancy phenomena, and also for specific word anxiety and general situational anxiety among stutterers. Situational anxiety cues would, for example, consist of size and type of audience, while specific word anxiety cues would comprise such elements as word meaning and the starting letters of words. But the question arises as to whether there are really two independent effects, and Wischner quotes a study by Shulman as evidence for this being the case. In this experiment stutterers were asked to read a different 500-word passage five successive times under each of two conditions to *E* alone and to an audience which was increased by one additional person for each successive reading. The first condition would clearly be that which was most favourable to adaptation effects. In fact adaptation occurred under both conditions, but was found to be greatest when the successive readings were made in unchanged circumstances, and Wischner suggests that this finding indicates that stuttering is a function of general situational anxiety.

Other experiments, Wischner states, provide evidence suggesting that specific word anxiety can be manipulated independently of general situational anxiety conditions.

However, Wischner conducts his own experiments to examine the influence of these two types of cue in a more precise way. In one experiment he employed two conditions, one where the same passage was read to the experimenter alone on 5 successive occasions, while in the other 5 different passages were read consecutively to E alone. The results for the first of these conditions showed a typical adaptation trend with stuttering showing a progressive reduction from first to fifth reading. The second condition provided an interesting deviation from expectation, showing a decrease in stuttering from first to second reading and a progressive increase from second to fifth reading. Both these observations from condition two (the drop and the rise in stuttering frequency) require explanation.

Wischner puts forward his tentative explanation of these latter results, arguing that the initial fall in stuttering represents the decrease in situational anxiety; the increase in stuttering from trial 2 to trial 5 he suggests is attributable to the progressive influence of powerful specific word anxiety. It is, however, difficult to see how specific word anxiety could assert itself in quite this variable way; a plateau following the second trial would have been more understandable in terms of Wischner's explanation.

Respecting direct experimentation upon manipulation of situational anxiety, Wischner quotes a study by Dixon (1947). Here the subjects read a different passage five times under each of three conditions; to E alone, to a group of 5 people, and over a telephone. The three conditions were held to be characterized by different degrees of situational anxiety for stutterers, with the telephone being most anxiety-provoking and the "experimenter alone" condition producing least effect on speech. In fact, perhaps for the reasons Wischner puts forward, the telephone produced less stuttering than the group situation. However, three different adaptation curves were derived for the three conditions and the data confirmed the notion that the height of the adaptation curve would, in this experiment, depend upon the degree of situational anxiety involved.

It is important, at this stage, to draw attention to an interesting feature of this particular experiment, namely that the degree of modification produced by adaptation is really quite modest; the adaptation curve has flattened out at a mean of 15 stuttered words on trial 4 compared with a mean of 22 on trial 1. In addition, it should be noted that the differences between situations are not great, varying between 22 and 30 words stuttered on trial 1 and between 15 and 17 on trial 5.

Having concluded that there is evidence for both an expectancy as well as an adaptation phenomenon, Wischner next considers whether there are any grounds for the existence of an *expectancy adaptation* phenomenon. In other words, is there a progressive reduction in *anticipated* stuttering as a function of repeatedly viewing the same material? Wischner, in fact, found evidence that this expectancy adaptation effect seemed to be present to some degree when immediate re-reading was involved, although not when the successive readings were spaced 24 hours apart.*

In essence Wischner appears to be arguing that his experiments, and those of some other workers, are consistent with a learning theory explanation concerning the origin and maintenance of stuttering. The paradigm is that certain cues, either general situational or word specific, have acquired the capacity to arouse anxiety and are thus productive of nonfluency. Because the reduction of anxiety follows closely upon the cessation of stuttering behaviour, the act of stuttering is reinforced, drive reduction ensuring the continuance of the stuttering pattern.

This theory clearly has attractive qualities and affords a sound and logically consistent account of some of the phenomena of stuttering. It is, however, less easy to see how this theory could account for one of the most compelling effects noted in connection with stuttering, namely the rhythm effect. One might also question whether drive reduction operates in the simple and direct manner suggested by Wischner. Is it possible that fluencies, which are generally greater in number than nonfluencies, might also be increased by drive reduction? Alternatively, if drive reduction operates differentially in favour of stuttering it is difficult to see why the stutterer should not become, at some stage, completely incapacitated.

However, the theory is sufficiently carefully worked, and backed by sound experimentation, and is capable of development to a stage where it has greater predictive power and greater coverage of facts than is presently the case.

* See Peins, 1961, 147.

6. *The Diagnosogenic Theory of Stuttering: Johnson*

This theory has an unusual feature as its starting point: namely, a denial that there is anything which one can reasonably call primary stuttering. The argument is that examples of nonfluencies are extremely common among young children, and that what we really need to explain is how nonfluencies persist in time and develop to a condition which we can legitimately call stuttering.

So far as can be seen the theory was first conceived out of the results of an inquiry into factors which it was thought might differentiate stutterers from nonstutterers. This inquiry was mainly concerned with the relative incidence in the two groups of difficult births, left-handedness, as well as other factors, and it seemed almost incidental to the main inquiry that a most important observation was made. The observation made was that it was extremely difficult to differentiate stutterers from nonstutterers on the basis of tape recordings of speech; both groups seemed to be characterized by a similar number of hesitations and repetitions.

This strongly suggested to Johnson that there were *in fact* no real differences between the groups, at least in terms of speech fluency, and that classification into "stutterer" and "nonstutterer" must have been made on some basis other than speech fluency.

To satisfy his curiosity about this apparent paradox Johnson began to ask the parents of stutterers about the early manifestations of speech difficulties in their child; to him these reports seemed to be concerned with the kinds of "normal" disfluency which one would expect to find in any child. From this point the theoretical argument was a simple one, containing three separate propositions. First, it seemed that whether a child was regarded as a stutterer depended upon the opinion of a lay person—most usually a parent; secondly, that the evidence on which stuttering was diagnosed concerned the kind of disfluencies found in every young child; and thirdly that "true" stuttering develops *after* the diagnosis has been made rather than before.

In short, a child who has been labelled a stutterer is likely to become worried about, and therefore focus attention upon, his speech in a way which is calculated to produce greater disruption rather than less. The implication behind this, however, is that the parent or whoever holds the responsibility for rearing the child, has an exaggerated concern for "correct" speech, has tended to attach undue significance to minor disfluencies, and has communicated this concern to the child. Johnson in fact hypothesized that the parents or guardians would be over-anxious and perfectionist and place greater emphasis upon unrealistically high expectations regarding cleanliness, politeness, etc.

Certainly work by Davis (1939, 1940a, b) is quoted as showing that nonfluencies are quite common among normal young children, although it is interesting to note that the characteristic letter or syllable repetitions of the "true" stutterer are rarely found. Other studies suggest that children who are regarded as "normal speaking" may be judged to stutter by persons instructed to listen for abnormalities in the tape-recorded speech of children.

Perhaps more convincing, however, is the finding that parents of stuttering children are *more likely* to diagnose stutters from recorded speech than are parents of nonstuttering children (Bloodstein *et al.*, 1952).* But even if this finding were confirmed by other studies it would not necessarily imply that stutters are *caused* by these high standards of parental expectation respecting speech. It may well be that parents of stutterers are, or have become, more aware of nonfluencies as a result of being exposed to them and being more concerned about them.

Further evidence for the link between parental sanctions and stuttering is contained in an unpublished study by Herbert (1966). In a study of children referred to a child guidance clinic in South Africa, Herbert found that the incidence of stuttering was much greater among children of Indian parents than those of African or white parents. Further inquiry revealed that cultural differences were strongly implicated, severe punishment for nonfluencies being far more common among the Indian community.

Moncur (1952) has also reported an investigation of parental attitudes in stuttering and nonstuttering groups. His findings suggest that stuttering is not related to any one specific environmental condition, but that there is some association between this disorder and problems concerning parental domination through disciplinary action, over-supervision of activities, over-critical or over-protective behaviour by parents, and setting unrealistically high standards in general.

However, in another study Goldman and Shames (1964a) report that no differences were found between parents of stutterers and nonstutterers in terms of goals which the parents set for themselves on

* See also Berlin, p. 38.

the Rotter Board (1942). Of course, while there may be an absence of differences in the personal standards of the two groups, it could well be that they differ in respect of the standards which they are prepared to impose upon others.

Accordingly, in a further study, Goldman and Shames (1964b) required the parents of stutterers and nonstutterers to estimate the future performance of their children on the Rotter Board as well as the degree of speech difficulty which their children might show on a story-telling task. It was found that the evidence supported the contention that the parents of stutterers set higher goals generally (as measured by the Rotter Board Test) and higher speech goals specifically (in terms of the story-telling task) than did parents of control subjects.

While this evidence might be considered suggestive of a causative role being played by parents in the acquisition of stutters, it is certainly not conclusive. Wingate (1959) was aware of this deficiency in the chain of Johnson's theoretical argument and set out to examine the general proposition that critical evaluation of nonfluency leads to the exacerbation of the difficulty. In doing so he points out that there already exists indirect evidence for the proposition, other than that quoted above. For example, requiring a stutterer to pay particular attention to the sound of his own voice, or subjecting him to some kind of stress, both seem to produce greater speech difficulty, while distraction appears to have the opposite effect. Further, Van Riper (1937) has shown that the threat of electric shocks as punishment for speech abnormalities markedly increases the severity of stutters, and Maddox (1938) has reported that stutterers are made worse by viewing themselves in a mirror.

Wingate's experiment compared simple interruption of stuttered speech, or signalling and recording the occurrence of stutters, with a control period without such interference. The experimental condition should, by calling the stutterer's attention to the abnormalities in no uncertain manner, make stutters more frequent. The opposite was found to be true, both the experimental "interruption" conditions producing improvement rather than deterioration in fluency.

Wingate explains these findings as showing that a "set to avoid stuttering" has been adopted and maintained. He feels that while it may be true that the stutterer will avoid certain words, situations, and the like, we cannot conclude that the stutter emerges from attempts to avoid nonfluency—indeed, Wingate argues, the evidence suggests that critical evaluation of speech is helpful in controlling the stutter.

A consideration of findings concerning the proposition that non-fluency is caused by attempts to avoid speech difficulty leads Wingate to attempt to formulate his own theory. He suggests that the stutterer's basic motivation is to maintain communication, based upon a "deep need" for interpersonal relations. (It should be noted that there is no real evidence for this, and the proposition has the status of an unsubstantiated assumption.) He goes on to argue that stuttering is learned and maintained because it is just as successful as fluent speech in securing communicative contact with the listener, and adds that the speech difficulty may even have the additional advantage of gaining sympathy and greater attention for the speaker.

In developing his thesis Wingate turns his attention to the type of learning theory model deriving from Johnson's theory. It is pointed out that Wischner likens stuttering to an instrumental avoidance response where the cue for avoidance might be a word or speech situation, the punishment is disapproval, and stuttering is the avoidant response. Wingate argues that stuttering does not avoid punishment and we really need to account for its persistence in spite of the punishing consequences. Also, while Wischner's original theory deals with anticipatory unpleasantness it fails to account for that which occurs during the act of stuttering.

Wischner's later formulation, according to Wingate, does provide a satisfactory explanation of the unpleasantness experienced during the act of stuttering. This modified account supposes that the tension level is raised, during communication, to the point where a "block" occurs and that efforts to overcome this "block" result in stuttering. Following a resumption of fluency, tension is reduced and stuttering is perceived as instrumental in securing release from tension; this sequence reinforces stuttering and ensures its persistence.

Johnson's theory is clearly an important one and has an obvious appeal in terms of the kind of facts with which it deals. The merits of Johnson's theory are obvious and the interest which it has aroused has been the impetus to much research and development. In particular, the theory has the great advantage of being derived from empirical research, a feature which tends to ensure that it is closely tied to observation and avoids the esoteric quality of some alternative models.

The evidence upon which the theory is based is fairly compelling and would be difficult to account for in terms of propositions other than those put forward by Johnson. The evidence is not always directly favourable to Johnson's theory, but much of it continues to be consistent with the kind of model proposed. For example, in a recent Russian study it was reported that while, for pre-school children, talking when alone produced no significant increase in skill, there seemed to be a progressively greater difference between talking alone and talking with others present with increases in age (Razdolsky, 1965). This suggests that, in general, increasing awareness of the implications of stutters for the listener is an important element in the disorder.

This theory, like all others currently formulated in connection with stuttering, requires further research and development, particularly as the basic assumptions of the theory (e.g. that the first nonfluencies of "stutterers" and nonstutterers are not differentiated, and that the former have a history featuring stress on fluency) are sometimes questioned in the light of all the evidence (Wingate, 1962a, b, c). However, the theory still appears to have some promise and continues to receive a good measure of support from those engaged in the field of stuttering.

7. *A Conflict Theory of Stuttering: Sheehan*

The basis of this theory is similar to that involved in certain other formulations, namely that the stutterer anticipates difficulty in articulation and his efforts to grapple with speech are themselves the stimulus to stutter. In other words, anxious preparation for speech ensures the occurrence of nonfluency.

There are five main points of evidence which Sheehan (1958b) considers important to the formulation of his model:

1. The frequently reported observation that stutterers are able to predict and anticipate their difficulties.

2. That "blocks" appear to occur in connection with the same sounds or words, i.e. the nonfluency is to some degree systematic.

3. That past experience of difficulty with certain words or situations has, or appears to have, an effect upon stuttering behaviour which will occur in the future.

4. That stress, e.g. the threat of electric shocks for nonfluency, exacerbates stuttering.

5. That situations which are calculated to reduce anxiety are associated with a reduction in stuttering.

Sheehan recognizes that the kind of nonfluencies exhibited by the confirmed stutterer might bear little resemblance to their presumed origin—the nonfluencies of the young child. The changes which have been introduced, which are largely tricks of speech or speech avoidance, are, for Sheehan, the result of interference by outside agencies, for example excessive parental emphasis upon fluency.

According to this theorist we need to offer explanations of two main phenomena; first, how it is that the "block" occurs at all, and secondly, how the release from "blocking" is achieved. The model which Sheehan offers to account for these phenomena is a more or less direct adaptation of Miller's double-approach—avoidance paradigm, and two main propositions are involved; first, that stuttering begins when conflicting speech approach and speech-avoidance tendencies reach equilibrium, and secondly, that during the block "fear-motivated avoidance" is reduced and release from the block is effected.

The conflict, states Sheehan, is both between speaking and not speaking as well as between being silent and not silent. The stutterer wants to speak but is ashamed to do so; wants to be silent but feels frustrated and guilty should he be so. In other words, stuttering is the result of a conflict between speech and silence, and avoidance is rooted in the competition between these tendencies.

The equilibrium between these forces or tendencies for speech and silence produces "blocking", but the balance of forces does not remain equal for long; either the approach tendency increases in strength or the avoidance tendency for speech is weakened. Sheehan argues that the stutter itself is strongly implicated as the agent which effects release from the "block", and that it probably does so by reducing the very "fear motivated avoidance" which produced the "block". The argument that the stutter serves to reduce fear involves three assumed "causes":

1. It is said that much of the fear experienced by the stutterer stems from attempts to hide the lack of fluency. During the "block" the stutterer is forced to abandon his struggle to conceal his difficulty and this removes part of his burden of fear.

2. To some extent the stutterer is the victim of a sense of helplessness and "fear of the unknown". Having the stutter occur is to

some extent reassuring as it places the abnormality in more real and less frightening perspective.

3. In line with Fenichel's hypothesis (1945) Sheehan argues that stuttering could be an aggressive act and the act of stuttering serves to temporarily reduce the need for aggression.

Certain obvious deductions may be derived from a conflict view of stuttering, both in terms of conditions which lead to decreases as well as those which produce increases in the abnormality. Stuttering should be made worse by increasing the avoidance drive (i.e. increasing the "penalty" for speech), or by decreasing the approach tendency, while reducing the avoidance tendency or increasing "approach" should effect an improvement in fluency. Sheehan claims that the results of experiments which have been concerned with the manipulation of these opposing drives or tendencies lend support to the theory.

In one such experiment Van Riper (1937) examined the influence of the threat of electric shock upon stuttering and found that stuttering frequency was increased. In another experiment, this time by Porter (1939), the effects of size and personnel of audience were investigated, and Sheehan claims that the results were consistent with the hypothesis that social penalty effects increases in stuttering behaviour.

Experiments which, in Sheehan's opinion, bear upon the problem by *reducing* the avoidance drive have also produced results which are consistent with the theory. In one study, by Eisenson and Horowitz (1945), it was found that the use of less meaningful material led to greater fluency, while the experiment by Eisenson and Wells (1942), concerning reduction in the degree of communicative responsibility, also affords support for Sheehan's position.

While several experiments are appropriate to the avoidance drive aspects of the model, Sheehan admits that experimental evidence for the effects of approach drive manipulation are lacking. In the latter case the evidence must be necessarily anecdotal, and Sheehan mentions situations such as halting requests for a raise in salary, or hesitant proposals of marriage as indicative of the effects of reduced approach drive. Strong approach tendencies may, however, produce remarkable fluency among stutterers (e.g. in crises).

Perhaps one of the most difficult aspects of Sheehan's theory concerns the proposition that stuttering reduces fear which, in turn, effects release from the block. He argues that demonstrations of the adaptation effect constitute supportive evidence for this; stuttering progressively reducing both the fear of stuttering and hence the tendency for nonfluencies to occur. Also, Sheehan quotes his own work, which involved continued repetition of a word until normal fluency was secured, as evidence consistent with a fear-reduction hypothesis.

However, he regards his experiment with Voas (1954) involving electromyographic readings from the masseter muscles of stutterers during the period of the block as constituting more direct and conclusive evidence. In this experiment the prediction was made that fear would increase as the stutterer moved through the block and so came closer to the feared goal of speaking. The results indicated that the greater tension, as shown by the electromyographic recordings, occurred just before release from the block which Sheehan regards as confirmation of the theory.

It is argued that the notion of the stutter as a fear-reducer clarifies the difficult point of why the avoidance of stuttering produces a build-up rather than a reduction of anxiety. When avoidance of stuttering can be achieved tension is increased, even though fluent speaking may be temporarily accomplished; when stutters occur, or the stutterer deliberately affects nonfluency, tension and anxiety are dissipated and greater fluency can be achieved as a result. Sheehan appears to be more satisfied by his attempt to resolve the paradox than seems to be justifiable. It is not easy to accept that fluent speech is storing up trouble for the stutterer if we also accept the proposition that fear and anxiety concerning stuttering precipitate the abnormality. However, the correctness of Sheehan's position is a matter for experiment and fact to decide rather than opinion.

Having postulated that stuttering produces fluency and fluency effects stuttering, Sheehan argues that we must draw a distinction between the fear reduction which occurs during the block and that which results after release. He goes on to say that sometimes the fear reduced after overcoming the block can be obscured by the fear which is aroused by nearing the goal of speaking. Apart from the great difficulty which might be experienced in attempting to disentangle these effects by experiment, it would be a most exacting task to demonstrate how the complex interactive processes involved combine to produce a particular outcome. Sheehan's theory must assume, however, that fear reduction which follows the block must either be greater than any fear increase which may "overlap" during the block, or that the former is in some way appreciably distinct from the latter. This is made necessary by his assumption that it is the state of lowered drive which follows release which serves to reinforce and perpetuate the behaviour pattern.

While, at this stage, no detailed account of the sources of conflict is essential, Sheehan offers some speculations concerning the nature and causes of the antagonistic tendencies which lead to stuttering behaviour. He believes that guilt is of prime importance as a source of conflict, which may be of two main kinds. First, there is the guilt which has led to the development of the stutter, and secondly that which is experienced because of the effect of the stutter upon the listener. The notion of heightened experience of guilt among stutterers receives little experimental support.* Guilt, according to the theory, can be reflected at various levels of conflict, for example at a level involving specific words, situations, or personal relationships. Conflict is also seen to occur at the "ego protective" level, and the desire to guard against experiences which are personally painful may, for example, lead the stutterer to avoid competitive situations.

This theory shares with certain others foundations which rest upon existing theoretical formulations, and which simply require the author of the theory to adapt the framework to his own special problem. Because of this such theories tend to have a somewhat *ad hoc* flavour and appear to have less promise than those which are based upon the observation of abnormalities; theories developed in one field must necessarily be under some degree of strain when applied to another field which is characterized by its own special problems.

Nevertheless, Sheehan's attempt to apply the concepts of conflict theory and research to stuttering behaviour has an obvious appeal, and the adaptation has been systematically developed. Certain aspects of the model fail to convince, however, especially the arguments involved and the experimental evidence adduced in support of the hypothesis that the stutter serves to reduce the fear which elicited the abnormality.

Naturally the most important consideration is that of whether or not Sheehan's theory generates experimentally verifiable deductions, and the extent to which these deductions are confirmed by critical test. In this respect a recent series of publications are of some interest.

Publications by Conway and Quarrington (1963) and by Quarrington

* However, see Sheehan, Cortese and Hadley (1962).

(1965) both drew conclusions in support of the theory of approach —avoidance gradients in stuttering. According to these authors the evidence suggests that such a theory would account not only for the within-phrase position gradient of stuttering difficulty (i.e. that words which occur earlier in the phrase are more likely to be stuttered), but also for the cyclic or wave-like manifestations of stuttering (i.e. the abnormalities of speech occur in clusters interspersed with fluent periods). However, a recent report by Taylor and Taylor (1966) re-examines the evidence for positional effects and "clustering" in stuttered speech. It is deduced from Sheehan's theory that the probability of stuttering any particular word in a phrase should increase as a function of prior fluency. In other words, as Sheehan argues that tension is produced by fluency, then stuttering should become more and more probable as the stutterer moves through the sentence. This deduction, as Taylor points out, is in conflict with the usually observed position gradient in which the first words of a sentence are more likely to be experienced as difficult, but the method of deriving this positional effect generally does not allow Sheehan's prediction to be tested as no account is taken of stutters which influence fluency. What is required to ensure adequate examination of Sheehan's hypothesis is to evaluate stuttering probability within phrases, given that no previous word in the phrase has been stuttered.

Taylor (1966b) provided data on 9 subjects and analysed only the first stutter in each phrase of the material read by the sample. With no prior stuttering events in any phrase, it was found that the probability of appearance of a nonfluency decreased as the phrase was read rather than increased as would be predicted from Sheehan's theory. Taylor and Taylor also re-examined the original data for 4 of the 9 subjects in the sample, this time to see whether or not the probability of stuttering was affected by a particular stuttering event. It will be recalled that Sheehan claims that his theory enables the prediction of "clustering" of stutters (although this is difficult to understand in view of his hypothesis that a stutter creates fluency), and the experiment by Taylor and Taylor set out to examine whether stutters are followed by fluency or by other stutters.

No probability trend was in fact discovered, either in support of the "clustering" hypothesis or the "fluency" prediction, and the results suggest no dependency between successive stuttering events.

Further research is clearly required before this theory, or parts of it, could be either accepted or rejected. Such research could be facilitated by an attempt to tighten-up the theory and so avoid certain ambiguities which it contains.

8. *Conclusions*

1. Theories of stuttering differ markedly in orientation and in the scope of the phenomena they seek to explain.

2. Although numerous theories exist concerning the aetiology and phenomena of stuttering none, as yet, provide a satisfactory explanatory framework.

3. Stuttering theories in general do not reflect the kind of progressive change and refinement which one might expect to characterize a developing science.

4. Lack of a hard core of established "facts" concerning stuttering phenomena give rise to doubts as to whether a satisfactory theory can be formulated at this stage.

CHAPTER 4

THE GENETIC AND ORGANIC FACTORS IN STUTTERING

Two main viewpoints have been expressed in the literature on stuttering. One of these appears to involve the emphasis upon stuttering phenomena as an extension and elaboration of normal characteristics, the difference between stutterers and others being merely quantitative, while the other involves notions of qualitative differences. Among the latter both personality and physical/constitutional factors have been reported.

In this chapter the evidence for the existence of physical/constitutional differences between stutterers and nonstutterers is examined under somewhat arbitrary but convenient headings.

1. *Laterality*

Perhaps one of the most widely held beliefs about stuttering is that it can occur when a naturally left-handed child is made to give preference to his right hand. This belief stemmed originally from uncontrolled observation, but when more became known about the functioning of the brain the theory of the "dominant gradient" was used to explain it. The theory argues that if one hemisphere of the brain is definitely dominant then the child reads and writes normally; on the other hand, if there is lack or weakness of dominance, confusion of hemisphere control may lead the child to read and write at times in "mirror fashion". This idea was elaborated by Orton (1928) who proposed that stuttering results from "comparable difficulties".

In the 1930's Travis and his associates developed Orton's idea into a more detailed theoretical explanation concerning the organic origin of stuttering, and this attracted great interest. It was hypothesized that speech is initiated or controlled by one side of the brain, usually the left, and the average person is right-handed. The stutterer is, however, neither definitely left-brained nor right-brained and, as a result, is often left-handed or ambidextrous. In addition to this, speech involved the co-ordination of muscles by both sides of the brain, but lack of complete dominance results in inco-ordination of these muscles and, hence, stuttering. If the child is left-handed and is forced to become right-handed, whatever cerebral dominance exists becomes disturbed and the confusion or conflict between the two halves of the brain results in stuttering. It should be noted that Travis abandoned this theory in the 1940's for lack of supporting evidence, but a belief in the relationship between laterality and stuttering is still common.

Positive evidence for the above propositions is found in several studies by Bryngelson (1935, 1940), and Bryngelson and Rutherford (1937). In these studies the emphasis was on showing that stutterers were more likely to be ambidextrous and more likely to have shifted handedness from left to right than the nonstutterers. The results obtained were consistently in favour of these hypotheses, in some cases four times as much ambidexterity and eight times as much shifting of handedness was found among the stutterers compared with the controls.

On the other hand, negative findings are reported in studies by Heltman (1940), Spadino (1941) and Van Dusen (1939) among others, who failed to find any differences between the groups. In a more recent study by Andrews and Harris (1964) no differences whatever were found in the distributions of handedness between their stuttering and nonstuttering children.

A somewhat more sophisticated method for establishing lack of cerebral dominance has been to examine the electroencephalographic (EEG) records of stutterers and nonstutterers (e.g. Douglass 1943; Rheinberger et al., 1943; Lindsley, 1940). In 1938 Raney had noticed a "tendency for there to be a greater percentage in amplitude of alpha activity on the nondominant side of the head" (p. 36). Following this Lindsley reported a trend for unilateral blocking of the alpha rhythm in the left occipital region to occur in right-handed children, and to occur in the right occipital region in left-handed children. He suggested that this finding supported the notion of some relationship between bilateral differences in cortical functioning and handedness. Similar differences in occipital EEG records for stutterers and non-stutterers were found by Douglass. However, when examining the records for the whole of each cerebral hemisphere, both Lindsley and Douglass failed to confirm Raney's findings. In addition, when

Rheinberger *et al.* matched children in terms of handedness it was found that nothing in the EEG records discriminated the stutterers from the nonstutterers.

Other studies reporting the use of EEG records in the investigation of stuttering are dealt with in another part of this chapter, but it may be seen that the popular belief that ambidexterity is found more often in stutterers than in nonstutterers, and that this is a sign of weakness of cerebral dominance, is based upon very slender evidence. The most viable explanation of the conflicting evidence is that tests of handedness are unreliable and often very subjective. As Penfield and Roberts (1959) have noted, "A number of investigators have pointed out that the greater the number of tests used, the fewer become the purely left- or right-handed." Others have sought to establish the existence of lack of cerebral dominance by more direct methods. A test of cerebral dominance which has not yet been fully investigated with stutterers is the phi-test.

The phi-phenomenon occurs when two lights are switched on and off in rapid succession until a point is reached when the alternation produces the effect of apparent movement of a single point of light. By presenting the two lights in a certain position in relation to each other, Jasper (1932) found that the direction in which the light was perceived to move indicated the dominant hemisphere of that person. Jasper had reported that there was evidence in his study which enabled him to "classify the stutterers quite definitely with the ambidextrous or left-handed groups of normal speakers" (p. 166). However, he wondered why certain ambidextrous persons did not stutter and why a few of the stutterers were more right-handed than the nonstutterers. He suggested that this test of central dominance in perception might be worthwhile pursuing further because it showed that the stutterers were practically 100% ambilateral. Raney (1935, 1938) has done further work on the test and the results show that in "normals" perceptual dominance does not always correlate with hand or eye dominance and may be a more reliable test of cerebral dominance than that of the culturally influenced handedness tests. Jasper's results are certainly of considerable interest and require replication and extension.

In recent years a very different test for establishing the cerebral dominance of an individual has been described by Wada and Rasmussen (1960). This is the intracarotid amytal test and involves the injection of sodium amytal into the carotid artery. While the

injection is in progress the patient counts and makes rapid alternating movements of the fingers of both hands. If the injection has
been given on the side of the non-dominant hemisphere the patient
will stop counting for a moment and then begin again and there
will be hemiplegia for about 5 minutes. If the dominant hemisphere
is involved, the patient will stop counting for a minute or so and then
be confused in his counting and have difficulty naming objects and
reading.

This test has been used in a very recent study by Jones (1966). He
had four stutterers with brain lesions in what were presumed to be
"speech areas" and who were severe and life-long stutterers. Jones,
like Jasper, found evidence for substantial bilateral representation
of speech, the stutterers developing aphasia when injected on both
the right *and* left side. Another most interesting feature of this report
is that all four stutterers stopped stuttering after their brain operation
and at this time the sodium amytal test produced aphasia only on
the side not operated upon. Jones says that "this indicates a transfer
of influence to one hemisphere only" and that the result suggests
"interference by one hemisphere with the speech performance of the
other" (p. 195).

This study must rekindle interest in the Travis theory.

2. *The Genetics of Stuttering*

The general feeling among most authorities on stuttering is that
one is more likely to find stutterers in the families of stutterers than
in the families of nonstutterers. The problem is to decide whether
this is due to the transmission of certain defective genes, to the
personal contact the child has with members of his family who stutter
or expect him to stutter, to the psychological atmosphere of the
home environment, or to a combination of any two or all three
influences.

One of the common methods employed to unravel the genetic from
the environmental effect is to study the occurrence of the particular
characteristic among twins. It is argued that if a genetic factor were
playing a dominant part in the appearance of stuttering then both
members of a pair of identical twins would be expected to stutter
more often than would a pair of fraternal twins. Evidence against
this being the case has been offered by Luchsinger (1940) and by
Graf (1955). Graf, for example, carried out a very extensive survey

among 85,680 American public school pupils. Among this sample were 552 pairs of twins and of these 21 individuals stuttered. A breakdown of these individuals showed there was one identical pair and two fraternal pairs in which both twins stuttered. These 21 stutterers comprised 1·90% of the twin sample.

Other evidence has been provided by Seeman (1939) who reported that both twins were more likely to stutter if they were identical. Similarly, Nelson et al. (1945) found that when stuttering occurred in identical twins then both members stuttered in all cases but one, and when it occurred among fraternal twins only one member of the pair stuttered in all cases except two. It is interesting to note that they also found that stuttering occurred in 20% of their 200 pairs of twins in contrast to the general expectation of about 1% and this may be viewed as support for Berry's contention (1938) that stuttering occurs more frequently in families with twins than in those without, as he reported stuttering expectancy in twinning families to be 1 in 18 (5·6%). On the other hand, Andrews and Harris failed to find such an association in their English study which is in agreement with Graf's report.

On the basis of the information given it is difficult to account for the discrepant results concerning the concordance of stuttering in identical twins. One hypothesis is that the discrepancy might result from inadequate methods for identifying whether a particular twin pair results from the division of a single fertilized cell or the coincident fertilization of two separate cells.

Perhaps the expectation itself is in doubt as many people have observed that, in identical twins, one is often right-handed and the other left-handed. For example, Newman et al. (1937) found that 16% of their twin pairs showed clear reversed handedness and 10% had one right-handed twin and the other ambidextrous. When reared apart Newman et al. reported that 11 out of 20 pairs showed reversed handedness.

The tendency for left-handedness or ambidexterity to be linked with cerebral dominance has not been firmly established but Raney (1938) thought that if there *were* a tendency for reversed lateral dominance in identical twins, this might appear on the phi-test which was mentioned in the previous section of this chapter. He gave the test to 17 pairs of twins and found that 88% showed reversed laterality. On the basis of this result one could well argue that concordance for stuttering in identical twins would be unlikely.

West *et al.* (1939) attempted to separate out stuttering which resulted from association with another stutterer and that which was genetically determined. They carefully matched 204 stutterers and nonstutterers and some of their data obtained are presented in Table 6.

TABLE 6

Table to show number of stutterers in the families of stutterers and controls and the number having associations with stutterers (West *et al.*, 1939)

	Stutterers	Controls
Number of stutterers in the families	210	37
Number of stuttering parents or grandparents	54	4
Number having no association with other stutterers	129	144
Number associating with other stutterers	75	60

These results obtained by West *et al.* would suggest that association with other stutterers is not an important factor in determining the development of stuttering, whereas it does seem to be important whether one has a stutterer in the family or not. Similar results to these have also been reported by Wepman (1939). In the West survey mentioned above, there was also evidence for a tendency toward sexual transmission of stuttering, in one group of families the females tended to be the stutterers while in another the males were affected.

Andrews and Harris (1964) point out that a lot of information has been lost in these studies because of the lack of modern genetic statistical techniques, for example, there is no breakdown of the data to show the frequency of stuttering among the parents and sibs. In their own survey they found a significant tendency for an increased risk of stuttering in the families of stutterers, thus supporting the conclusions of both Wepman and West *et al.* They suggest that this is not due to imitation or learning on the part of the child because only 20% of their cases had any close contact with another stutterer. They also hypothesize that sex-limitation is an operative factor in the transmission of stuttering. That is to say, there are certain genes of the female that act so as to modify the effect of the "stuttering" gene(s). They are also of the opinion that transmission may be "by a common dominant gene with a multifactorial background. . . . Alternatively, inheritance may be wholly polygenic" (p. 143).

The existing evidence seems to suggest that some hereditary factors may be operating in the development of stuttering, but the method of transmission is uncertain as is the degree to which it can be, and is, modified by environmental factors. It may be something in the nature of a predisposition to faulty speech which is inherited and that the development of florid stuttering depends on whether such factors as those described by Johnson (see Chapter 3) are operative in the environment. Arguments evoking the notion of predisposition have little or no explanatory value unless there is some way of describing accurately the predisposing mechanism. If, for instance, the phi-test or the sodium amytal test could be given to all children who have a family history of stuttering, then predictions could be made as to which child was predisposed to develop a stutter and which not. In such a case the notion of predisposing factors becomes of great value both from the theoretical and practical point of view.

3. *The Cardiovascular System*

Little has been written concerning the relationship between stuttering and properties of the blood and functions of the heart. Karlin and Sobel (1940) found no differences in blood patterns between two matched groups of stutterers and nonstutterers and they question the statistical procedures used by previous workers. For example, Kopp (1934) found stutterers to have a higher calcium and phosphorus content in the blood, but the stutterers were younger than the normals. Also, on recalculating the data and using a two-tail instead of a one-tail test of significance, four out of the five differences found were not significant. Anderson and Whealdon (1941) could find no differences in the distribution of blood groups between stutterers and 38,000 United States control nonstutterers.

While Ritzman (1943) failed to find significant differences in heart rate between stutterers and nonstutterers, Travis *et al.* (1936) reported that all the stutterers in their sample showed tremors of about 10 seconds on an electrocardiogram. Their results, however, led them to conclude that any changes in heart rate that occurred during speech were secondary to changes in respiration and general body activity, and that this applied to both stutterers and nonstutterers.

However, they report that varied and striking changes in the heart functioning do occur during severe stuttering.

Allergic reactions are held by many to be the result of, among other things, a disturbance of the cardiovascular system and the autonomic nervous system, and both Card (1939) and Kennedy and Williams (1938) have reported results suggesting a causal relationship between allergic reactions and stuttering. Card, for example, has reported that 102 of 104 stutterers had allergies either themselves or in their families, compared with 62% of a nonstuttering group.

Kennedy and Williams (1938) interviewed the parents of 100 stuttering children and found that 95 out of the 100 had a personal or family history of allergy, 52 of them having a personal history of an allergic reaction. They cite as a control sample a previous study of 1000 people of whom 28% had a family history and under 2% had a personal history only. From these data they suggest the existence of a close association between allergic manifestations and stuttering leading to the assumption of "a cerebral cortex which is hypersensitive to any transient vasomotor disturbance brought about not by a specific allergen but by the effort of speech" (p. 1308).

Thus, both these studies report very high correlations indeed between the presence of allergies and stuttering compared with non-stutterers. The main difficulty in evaluating these results is that the investigators themselves took the case histories with the full knowledge of the aim of the project, and the essentially subjective procedure of taking a case history is very prone to the influence of bias on the part of the experimenter. One might also expect that if such a clear-cut relationship existed, then other research workers might have been struck by the number of stutterers with allergic symptoms. An interesting incidental finding by Card, which does not appear to have been followed up, is that stuttering ceased after an injection of adrenalin.

4. *Metabolism and Physiology*

In 1934 Kopp concluded that "stuttering is a manifestation of a disturbed metabolism". He found that the total serum calcium inorganic phosphate and blood sugar were significantly higher in stutterers than in nonstutterers, while the total protein, albumin and globulin were significantly lower. Previously, in 1933, Johnson *et al.* had reported serum calcium and potassium to be *normal* in stutterers as was their carbohydrate metabolism. However, as mentioned on p. 86, these findings of Kopp are in doubt. In a review of this early literature, Hill (1944) came to the conclusion that there was no evidence for an abnormally high level of serum calcium in stutterers.

Several people have suggested that stuttering is a form of latent tetany, in particular West (1958) and Johnson et al. (1959) argue that in latent tetany the serum calcium in the body remains just above a critical level. Although they point out that there is no evidence for this being the case they say that hyperventilation may also lead to tetany. Overbreathing has been reported to impair the motor performance of nonstutterers (Lillehei and Balke, 1955; Rahn et al., 1946) and to be accompanied by a drop in alveolar carbon dioxide. They then argue that moderate hyperventilation could produce an increase in stuttering in the stutterer. No such effect was in fact found. However, they do report a slight decrease in the speech fluency of the nonstutterers after hyperventilation and reason that this constitutes further suggestive evidence that stuttering should be differentiated from the nonfluency of normal speakers.

A reduced hydrogen ion concentration in conjunction with reduced carbon dioxide tension has also been a supposed causal factor in hyperventilation tetany. Both Kelly (1932) and Starr (1928) have reported the hydrogen ion concentration to be high in stutterers resulting in pH values below those for normal individuals. (A hydrogen ion is an atom of hydrogen bearing a single positive electric charge.) Both authors interpret this as meaning that the stutterer has a considerable amount of carbon dioxide present in the blood due to inefficient breathing. Starr later confirmed his findings and stressed that stutterers have characteristically high alveolar carbon dioxide. The results obtained by Johnson et al. (1959) contradict this assumption since the infrared carbon dioxide analysis employed by them is purported to produce similar results to those derived from blood analyses.

Whether stutterers do or do not have more carbon dioxide in their blood than normal speakers remains in doubt, but this has not prevented some clinicians from using the gas as a therapeutic device.

The use of carbon dioxide (CO_2) in the treatment of the neuroses was pioneered by Meduna (1950). Smith (1953) also administered this gas to 33 stutterers three times a week and reported that 11 of these improved 100%, 3 improved 75%, 2 improved 50%, 5 improved 25%

and 12 showed no improvement. He concludes that speech clinicians generally fail to achieve comparable results and recommends that stutterers should be treated by the psychiatrist using carbon dioxide.

On the other hand, Arthurs et al. (1954) have attempted to replicate Smith's work using a modification of the procedure. They used nitrous oxide up to the point of light anaesthesia and then carbon dioxide. Using objective measures of stuttering frequency and expert ratings of severity, they report a failure to find any improvement in fluency as a result of the treatment.

In this connection it is of some interest to note that Kent (1961) reports the results of a poll taken from members of the Carbon Dioxide Association to find out whether any of them now used carbon dioxide in the treatment of stuttering. Her conclusions, on the basis of replies received, were that "the efficacy of this treatment for stuttering has not been answered adequately either through research or through the experiences of clinicians" (p. 271). She also comments that an interesting sidelight gleaned from the correspondence is that several members noted that the success of the treatment seemed to depend upon the age at which stuttering started. Cases which begin to stutter in adolescence or later seem to do better with the treatment than cases with a history of earlier onset.

A different approach to the study of metabolism in stutterers has been made by McCrosky (1957). He found no difference in the basal metabolic rate (the measure of total heat production over a given period of time during the post-absorptive state) between stutterers and nonstutterers in the speaking and nonspeaking situation. The

TABLE 7

Means, percentages, and standard deviations for BMR, SMR, and PSMR of stutterers and nonstutterers (McCrosky, 1957)

	Nonstutterers	Stutterers
Mean BMR (%)	−15·12	−14·17
SD	5·76	14·21
Mean SMR (%)	− 3·87	− 2·63
SD	8·43	15·97
Mean PSMR (%)	−10·69	− 8·11
SD	5·61	9·78

rate was, however, significantly higher for both groups during the latter condition. The means and standard deviations for the basal metabolic rate (BMR), the speech metabolic rate (SMR) and the post-speech metabolic rate (PSMR) are shown in Table 7. This demonstrates, very clearly, the great variation obtained on a measure *within* a group of stutterers, even in something as fundamental as the basal metabolic rate.

McCrosky looked to see if there might be two classes of stutterer, which would explain the lack of significant differences in their scores compared with nonstutterers. He divided his group into those who were receiving treatment and those who had completed treatment, finding that the mean SMR for the post-treatment group was $-8 \cdot 77$ and for the current treatment group $+11 \cdot 96$ ($p < 0 \cdot 01$). This must probably be one of the factors contributing to the very large standard deviations shown in Table 7. The post-treatment group also had a significantly ($p < 0 \cdot 05$) smaller difference between their basal and speech metabolic rates compared with the current treatment group, but they did not differ in this respect from nonstutterers.

By breaking down the stutterer group into two sub-groups in a meaningful way, McCrosky was able to show how some of the very large variation in scores could be accounted for. He did not reanalyse the whole of his data in terms of these two groups and so his conclusion that "There is no significant difference between the stutterer and the nonstutterer with respect to basal metabolic rate" (p. 51) must stand.

In a single case study, Stratton (1924) has produced evidence suggesting that the urinary creatinine coefficient of the sub-breathing stutterer is lower than in the normal breather on a similar diet. He also found that an increase in stuttering is preceded by a decrease of creatinine in the urine and vice versa. He concludes by saying that "If urinary creatinine coefficient is low in sub-breathing stammerers then it may be concluded that faulty metabolism is an important factor in the etiology of stammering and must therefore be corrected to effect a cure." Unfortunately there does not appear to have been any follow-up of this finding on a group of stutterers.

One of the earliest reports of a possible relationship between stuttering and endocrine malfunctioning (Gordon, 1928) concerned the appearance of stuttering speech in five cases who were given thyroid extract to counteract a thyroid deficiency. Stuttering disappeared when the extract was stopped. Following on this Glaser

(1936) sent questionnaires to 35 prominent endocrinologists seeking their observations on the development of stuttering during the course of endocrine therapy. The general conclusion was that no evidence existed to suggest a casual relationship of the kind postulated, but 6 of the 35 experts did report having observed an association in such disturbances as hyperinsulinism and thyroid insufficiency.

A possible clarification of whether there is some connection between stuttering and endocrine malfunction is offered by Cabanas (1954). His investigation concerned the study of 50 mongoloid children when they were receiving and when not receiving thyroid extract. He reported that certain abnormalities of speech were observable of a "cluttering type", but thought it possible to differentiate this hurried speech, with its hesitations, blockings and repetitions, from stuttering, because there was no associated attempts at avoidance, and no word fears or associated body movements. Although the picture is far from clear it may be that the "stuttering" observed by other writers was in fact the "cluttering" resulting from hurried speech observed by Cabanas. Since no generally accepted definition of stuttering speech exists, it seems most important that accurate quantification be made of the type of speech abnormalities observed, so that direct comparisons across studies can be carried out. Until this is achieved the use of the term "stuttering" for any "stuttering-type" behaviour can only continue adding to the confusion that already exists.

5. *Drugs*

The effects of a drug and/or placebo on the stutterer have been investigated both in the experimental situation and as a form of treatment. The group of drugs arousing the most interest in the treatment of stuttering in recent years has been the tranquillizers and the most popular of these have been reserpine, chlorpromazine and meprobamate.

The tranquillizer drugs have a calming effect without inducing sleep or obviously altering the state of consciousness. It is because they are more than a sedative that people have considered it worthwhile to continue investigating their effects on stuttering in spite of discouraging results from the use of sedatives. For instance, Love (1955), in a well-designed experiment using each subject as his own control, found no significant differences in stuttering frequency whether nembutal (a depressant), benzedrine (a stimulant), lactose (a placebo) or no drug was given before a subject read a passage of prose eight times. While the *t*-tests employed were an inappropriate statistic (in 28 out of 32 cases the standard deviation was greater than the mean), Fig. 7 shows quite clearly that the drugs had no differential influence upon stuttering. It is, however, interesting to note the consistently higher mean number of words stuttered for the placebo reading condition in this experiment.

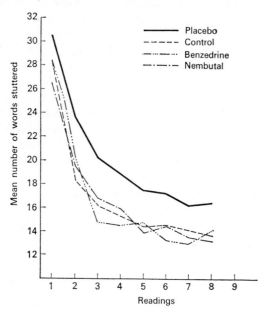

FIG. 7. Mean number of words stuttered during each of eight successive readings after the administration of benzedrine, nembutal, and placebo capsules, respectively, and in the control situation (Love, 1955).

Apparently different results were obtained by Palasek and Curtis (1960) as is shown in Fig. 8. Here the "no capsule" condition (*A*) produced a consistently (although not significantly) greater number of speech blocks than did the lactose condition (*D*). However, the two experiments are not directly comparable. Palasek and Curtis administered the capsules randomly and in such a way that neither the subject nor the experimenter knew the contents of any one capsule, but the first condition for *all* subjects was the control condition under which no capsule was administered. It would also appear that in this experiment the subjects read the *same* passage five times on each test day with 48 hours between each test; the authors state that "It was assumed that the spacing between conditions was sufficient to eliminate reductions of stuttering attributable to adaptation after the control reading. It is impossible, however, to state with any certainty that adaptation was not a factor" (p. 225).

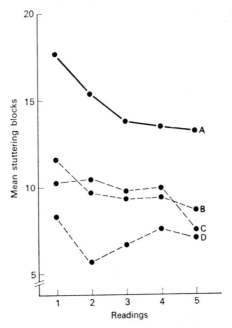

FIG. 8. Mean number of stuttering blocks for each of five readings in the control (no placebo) and experimental (placebos of lactose and calcium carbonate) conditions: A = control condition, B = 11 grains calcium carbonate, C = 5·5 grains lactose and 5·5 grains calcium carbonate, D = 11 grains lactose (Palasek and Curtis, 1960).

On the basis of the literature on the adaptation effect reported in Chapter 6 one must endorse this last statement. Love, on the other hand, had different reading material on each of the experimental days and included the control day in the randomization of conditions.

From the summary table of the analysis of variance provided by Palasek and Curtis, it is apparent that the main effect for subjects, and the subject interaction with readings and conditions, were all statistically significant. These data provide the explanation of why the differences in speech errors between the drug conditions plotted in Fig. 8 do not approach significance. This large variability among stutterers' responses to various experimental conditions is a constantly recurring theme throughout the literature.

Reserpine was the first of the tranquillizing agents to be used in the Western world and it was the first to be investigated in relation to stuttering. This involved a single case investigation by Meffert (1956) in which the male stutterer was given reserpine for 5 weeks, a placebo for 4 weeks, reserpine again for 4 weeks and finally reserpine plus speech therapy for 6 weeks. A reduction was found in the amount of stuttering manifested in both reading and conversation whenever the drug was being given, and an increase in stuttering when the placebo was administered.

Group data on the effects of reserpine have been obtained by other workers. Mitchell (1955), for example, treated 16 stutterers on a schedule of 4 weeks reserpine, 3 weeks no treatment and 4 weeks placebo. Eight of the stutterers received the conditions in the order, drug: no treatment: placebo: and 8 in the order, placebo: no treatment: drug. The results of this experiment showed no significant changes in severity of stuttering when the conditions were presented in this way. In both Meffert's and Mitchell's studies the stutterers gave subjective reports of improved attitudes towards their stuttering together with a decrease in anxiety. In another study by Hollister (1955), out of 6 stutterers treated for 30 days on reserpine and 30 days on placebo, both with speech therapy, 2 were found to be unchanged, 2 to have improved only when on reserpine, 1 only improved when on placebo, and 1 improved when on either reserpine or placebo.

In a paper discussing the use of tranquillizers in the treatment of stuttering, Kent (1963) cites two personal communications. One of these was from Heaver, Franklin and Arnold who gave to 4 groups of 10 stutterers either reserpine, reserpine–placebo, chlorpromazine or chlorpromazine–placebo over a period of 9 weeks. They reported that the drug groups could not be differentiated from the placebo groups on the speech measures which they used. The other communication was from Glasner who had used reserpine in the treatment of severe child stutterers. No objective measures were used but his subjective impressions were that the children were more relaxed and quieter generally under the drug, although only a few showed improvement in speech. He reported a similar increase in relaxation and greater spontaneity of speech in adults but was "less inclined to recommend the use of drugs than formerly".

There seems very little evidence on which to base the conclusion that reserpine has any effect upon the frequency of stuttering in adults or children, but the findings do suggest that the individual seems to respond to the drug by becoming less anxious and generally calmer, and this may be of value to some stutterers.

Hackett *et al.* (1958) studied the effects of another tranquillizer (chlorpromazine) in conjunction with speech therapy on the speech of child stutterers. All the children received a placebo for 6 weeks in the first instance, and were then given chlorpromazine for a further 6 weeks. After 12 weeks the children were divided into two subgroups, one having the drug and the other having the placebo for another 24 weeks. At the end of this time the authors report that the drug played a significant part in the speech improvement which occurred in over 80% of the active drug group, whereas in the placebo group only just over 30% showed similar improvement. In addition it was noted that the drug group tended to maintain its improvement in speech a year later whereas the placebo group had tended to relapse.

Chlorpromazine was also used by Winkelman (1954) in a study of 142 neuropsychiatric patients, of whom 5 were stutterers. The improvement in the speech of these five patients while on this drug ranged from marked improvement to no improvement. Kent (1963) notes that Winkelman reported in a personal communication to her that the "improvement" ratings were based upon observed changes in general level of anxiety and in speech, and that no quantitative measures of anxiety or speech were used.

On the basis of the studies quoted, and that of Heaver *et al.* already mentioned, the conclusion might be drawn that the case for chlorpromazine being an aid to reducing frequency of stuttering is not as yet established. The clinical report of Winkelman cannot, for example, be properly assessed and of the two experiments, one employed child while the other used adult subjects. The picture is also complicated by the fact that the adults were receiving group psychotherapy and the children "expressive symptomatic therapy", the dosages were not comparable, and the methods of measurement were different. However, the evidence is suggestive of some positive "real" effect and should serve to prompt further investigations of the effect of chlorpromazine on stuttering.

Another tranquillizer used in the treatment of stutterers has been meprobamate. In one study Kent and Williams (1959) compared a group of college student stutterers receiving a placebo and a group receiving this drug. On the basis of data derived from four measures made before and after a 14-week period of treatment, it was concluded that the two groups did not differ in the degree of improvement obtained.

A study in which meprobamate was used *without* speech therapy was reported by Di Carlo *et al.* (1959). They randomly assigned 30 adult stutterers to a drug, placebo or no treatment group for an experimental period of 6 weeks. The reduction in the mean number of stutters in those having meprobamate was not significant at the 5% level of confidence, whereas the *increase* in stuttering for the placebo group *was* significant. There was no demonstrable change in stuttering frequency for the no-drug group.

Another investigation into the effects of meprobamate on stuttering without any accompanying speech therapy (Holliday, 1959) employed a group of 20 male stutterers subdivided into drug and placebo groups. Varous measures of stuttering behaviour were taken before and after the 3-week experimental period. No significant differences were found in the measures of frequency or duration of stuttering but a significant decrease in tension ratings made by two clinicians was observed.

It seems that the tranquillizer meprobamate has a similar effect on stutterers to that of chlorpromazine and reserpine in that the drug seems to exert a tension- and anxiety-reducing influence. However, there is no evidence that this drug has any direct effect upon the stutter itself.

6. *The Nervous System*

Several of the EEG studies of stutterers have already been mentioned in the section on laterality, but some additional investigations deserve mention.

Douglass (1943) found that there was a significantly higher percentage of alpha rhythm in the left hemisphere of stutterers ($p < 0.01$) than in the right hemisphere but noted that this was not the case for nonstutterers. This finding has been confirmed by Knott and Tjossem (1943), and by Lindsley (1940) who found that the alpha waves of the two cerebral hemispheres were out of phase more of the time in ambidextrous and left-handed stutterers than in right-handed stutterers. It was also reported that periods of asynchronism of the alpha waves could be observed preceding most stuttering episodes.

More recently, Knott *et al.* (1959) have investigated whether the EEG correlates of anxiety, which have been described by Ulett, would discriminate between stutterers and nonstutterers. They tested two groups of stutterers ($N=19$ and 24) using a flickering light as the stimulus. In this study a difference was found between the first group of stutterers and the nonstutterers, with the former showing similar alpha band activity to Ulett's "anxiety-prone" group. There was, however, no such difference between the second group of stutterers and the nonstutterers, indeed it was found that on other measures the two stutterer groups differed from each other more than either did from the nonstuttering group.

Andrews and Harris (1964) used the electroencephalograph to explore more fully the possibility of neurological abnormality in 30 pairs of children. No differences were found between the EEG records of the stuttering and nonstuttering children when they were interpreted by an expert who was not aware of the group identity of each record. Differences also failed to emerge when the records were sorted into stutterer/control pairs and a judge was asked to assess which appeared to be the more abnormal of the pair.

In another study Travis (1934) measured the action current potentials of the two masseter muscles. He found that the action potentials for these muscles on either side of the jaw were identical during normal speech, but that during stuttering one reacted in a strikingly different way from the other. He hypothesized that normally there was a unified control by the central nervous system of motor components during speech but that this unity broke down during stuttering.

Williams (1955) also studied the action potential of the masseter or main jaw muscle during stuttered and nonstuttered speech. He found no bilateral differences in amplitude or in the time at which the action current appeared, but did find significantly more "spiking" in the stutterers during moments of stuttering. This "spiking" phenomenon was also demonstrated, however, when the nonstutterers faked stuttering and Williams concluded that any anomalies that occurred were part of the peripheral motor activity involved in stuttering and were not related to some fundamental CNS disturbance.

Research on the optics of stutterers was carried out by Gardner (1937). He made numerous measures of pupillary responses to light during silence and during speech and the results led him to conclude that the balance between the constrictor and dilator muscles of the pupil is "disarranged" in the stutterer. He points out that it is not possible to state on the basis of his evidence whether this is due to a general disorganization throughout the nervous system or to the greater emotionality of the stutterer during speech.

There has been considerable interest in recent years in the relationship between delayed auditory feedback and stuttering. This literature has been reviewed in Chapter 7 of this book and it is sufficient to say here that since the publication of Lee's (1951) paper "Artificial stutter", there has been discussion of whether there may be some perceptual disturbance involving the central nervous system in stutterers. Some evidence to support this case has been offered by Stromsta (1956) and by Rousey et al. (1959), but a more direct test of the hypothesis that stutterers have a disorder of the auditory central nervous system has been carried out by Gregory (1964). His qualified conclusion was that his results do not support the hypothesis. The qualification concerned the fact that the stutterers gave consistently poorer performances on speech discrimination tests, although on only one in eight tests was this difference significant at the 1% level of confidence. This being so, Gregory suggests that the area should be investigated more thoroughly, particularly with young subjects as any difference which may exist could be more apparent nearer the age of the onset of stuttering.

Attention to the possible implications of defects in the auditory apparatus has also been paid by Shearer and Simmons (1965); no differences were found between a group of 5 stutterers and 5 non-stutterers in middle-ear muscle activity during vowel phonation, counting, whispering and unvoiced oral movements.

7. The Respiratory System

Much of the early work on the breathing patterns of stutterers was carried out in Germany at the turn of the century (e.g. Halle, 1900; Ten Cate, 1902; Gutzmann, 1912) and all recorded various disturbances and abnormalities. In 1927, Travis reported certain differences between the breathing of normal speakers and stutterers, one of which was that while the normal speaker has a fairly close correspondence between thoracic and abdominal breathing, the stutterer shows complete antagonism between the action of the thorax and abdomen. Differences between these groups were also noted in respect of the relationship between laryngeal and breathing movements.

Starr's (1922) investigation of the breathing of stutterers was one of the early demonstrations that stutterers cannot all be pressed into the same mould. In the case of breathing activity, Starr found that the stutterers could be divided up into four subgroups. The majority were "sub-breathers" who were described as "organisms overloaded with carbon dioxide". For such persons Starr advocated breathing exercises and a decrease in the carbohydrate content of the diet. The second group were called "psychopathic" which Starr defined as meaning hyperexcitable; this group he considered to be hopeless from the point of view of remedial measures. The third group were "sub-breathers" *and* "psychopathic", and the fourth just hyperexcitable. Of this last group Starr comments that "perhaps it is from this class that the psychoanalyst recruits his subjects".

In 1931 Blackburn reported stutterers to be defective in voluntary control of various muscle groups including movements of the diaphragm during speech. Seth (1934) confirmed the results concerning the abnormalities of diaphragm control but this time in the *non-speaking* situation, and concluded that "respiratory disturbance in the stuttering subject is not due to or induced by the social situation in which communication by speech is demanded of the sufferer".

Van Riper (1936) investigated the breathing abnormalities occurring not only during overt stuttering but also during the expectancy of stuttering and reported that the same type of breathing abnormality occurred in both situations. He found particularly that expectancy of stuttering tended to show itself in a high inspiration–expiration ratio, increased variability, and the appearance of breathing irregularities.

In another study, Downton (1955) compared the breathing of stutterers under four conditions, but no statistical procedures were used on the data nor are any figures quoted. One of the interesting observations made in this study, however, was that there was less irregularity in breathing when the stutterer was told to feel "perfectly free to perform his stuttering easily and loosely . . ." (p. 283) than when he was told to attempt to prevent the occurrence of stuttering.

Other people have reported abnormalities in the breathing of stutterers, among them have been Steer (1935) who found anomalies in the breathing of children, and Fossler (1930). The latter worker reported that stutterers showed 29% more variability than normals in the duration of inspiration and 27% more variability than normals in the duration of expiration. Fossler concluded that differences in the breathing patterns of stutterers and nonstutterers do exist but that there were very great individual differences between the patterns of breathing records of this group.

It seems probable from these studies that stutterers do manifest abnormalities of breathing, and the main problem is that of deciding whether stuttering is responsible for the appearance of these abnormalities or whether faulty breathing is responsible for stuttering.

Starbuck and Steer (1954) believed that it might be of value to investigate whether there is any evidence for systematic alteration in the breathing patterns of stutterers or nonstutterers during the course of adaptation. In their experiment a group of 22 male stutterers was matched with 22 male nonstutterers and all were given a 200-word passage to read 5 times during which time records of breathing were obtained. Ordinarily a decrease in stuttering or nonfluencies would be expected (adaptation) and this indeed occurred, as Starbuck and Steer have reported in a previous paper (1954). Changes in breathing were also observed to take place during the 5 readings but the *type* of change appeared to be different for each group. For the stutterers there was an overall reduction in the number of complete thoracic and abdominal breathing cycles, whereas the nonstutterers manifested an increase in the depth of thoracic inhalation and a decrease in the depth of abdominal inhalation and exhalation. Thus, increasing familiarity with a reading passage and the experimental situation is reflected in changes in patterns of breathing, but the type of change likely to occur appears to differ for the stutterer and the nonstutterer.

8. *The Muscle System*

Simon (1945) hypothesized that each individual has a particular "level of integration" and that this tends to be particularly low for people with certain atypical behaviours, including stutterers. On a series of tests he devised, stutterers showed a "disintegration of function", i.e. they were less able to deal with the more complex situations than the nonstutterers. However, Ross (1955) gave these tests to a group of stutterers and a group of nonstutterers who were carefully matched for age, sex and intelligence and failed to find any significant differences, except on a speed test in which the stutterers performed at a higher level. He attributed the lack of agreement between this outcome and Simon's results as being due to his more careful matching of the two groups.

Such contradictory results are common in the literature concerning investigations into the motor abilities of stutterers. On psycho-motor tasks, for example, Bills (1934) has reported that vocal and manual blocks were twice as long and twice as frequent in stutterers as in nonstutterers and that the former had greater irregularities in reaction times. Again, in a study of reaction times to word associations, Adams and Dietze (1965) found that the stutterers were significantly slower than the normal speaking controls on all the words used. Also Rotter (1955) found stutterers inferior to nonstutterers in a card-sorting task when using only the right or the left hand but not when both hands were used together. On the other hand, both Cross (1936) and Lightfoot (1948) failed to demonstrate any difference in the motor capacities of stutterers and nonstutterers.

Regarding manual skill, Westphal (1933) found no difference between child stutterers and nonstutterers in strength or in hand–eye co-ordination, but Bilto (1941) reported the former to be inferior. In speed of repetitive manual movement West (1929) reported stutterers inferior, but Rotter (1955) and Strother and Kriegman (1943) found no significant differences. Similar contradictions are to be found in respect of rhythmic movements of the hands and these are discussed in the section of rhythm (Chapter 7).

Two studies report the use of the Oseretsky Tests of Motor Proficiency (1931). In the first of these, Kopp (1943) investigated 450 stutterers to determine the extent of the relationship between stuttering and general motor disturbances. The majority of studies already cited have been able to find either no differences between stutterers and nonstutterers, or have found differences which are comparatively small, or else positive results have been contradicted by subsequent studies. In contrast to all these, Kopp was led to state on the basis of her findings that "these motor disturbances are so significant that reversing the classic proposition, we may say that stuttering is not a psychologic disorder; it is first and, above all, a neurologic disorder characterized by profound disturbance of the motor function" (p. 114). She also states that "Gross hereditary defects of the motor function and disturbances of various motor systems are almost invariably found among stutterers. They are especially manifest when stuttering is constitutional and they are still very distinct when stuttering is acquired" (p. 116).

So striking were Kopp's results that Finkelstein and Weisberger (1954) decided that the investigation should be repeated. Their subjects were 15 stutterers matched for age, sex and handedness with 15 nonstutterers. They found that their stutterers were slightly (but not significantly) *in advance* of the controls in motor age. When compared with the norms provided by Oseretsky, the stutterers were retarded 3·5 months on average and the nonstutterers 12·0 months.

One of the reasons offered by Finkelstein and Weisberger to account for these two grossly discrepant findings is that they used the English adaptation of the test (Doll, 1940), while Kopp used the original. Doll comments that the scoring standards for this test are rather subjective and ambiguous and this being the case then the bias of the tester becomes a potent variable.

A few studies have attempted to identify some differences in muscle control of the jaw, tongue and lips between stutterers and non-stutterers during speech. For instance, Strother and Kriegman (1943) reported stutterers to be superior (but not significantly so) on the rate of diadochokinetic movements of lips, jaw and tongue. However, even after pooling the results from previous studies no significant differences emerged.

In another study tongue strength was found to be equal in stutterers and nonstutterers (Palmer and Osborn, 1940). Contradictory results have been reported concerning the making of repetitive lip, tongue and jaw movements, Cross (1936) finding that stutterers were slower than nonstutterers, while Spriestersbach (1940) did not. Similarly, West (1929) reported his stutterers to be inferior in the rate of jaw and brow movements while Spriestersbach's did not. An early report by Blackburn (1931) stated that stutterers showed a particularly marked inferiority to nonstutterers in executing rhythmical voluntary movements of the tongue and diaphragm, and a similar report was made by Hunsley (1937). Such differences were not, however, found by Seth (1934) or by Strother and Kriegman (1944).

Little seems to have been done concerning the eye movements of stutterers since a small number of reports were published in the 1930's. Murray was one of the first in the field to record the eye movements of stutterers during silent reading and compared these with a group of normal speakers. He found that stutterers had an average of $22 \cdot 34\%$ more fixations per line and $126 \cdot 5\%$ more "regressive" movements. In addition to this the stutterers were about one "grade" below the normal in comprehension of what they read, and two "grades" below in rate of reading (1932).

Jasper and Murray (1932) carried out the same kind of investigation of eye movements during oral reading. They report similar findings, i.e. the stutterers employed more fixations and regressive movements per line. This finding was subsequently also supported by Moser (1938). In his study there were also greater differences shown by the stutterers between silent and oral reading on all measures used. Moser added other evidence showing that none of his 52 stutterers were able to fixate a dot continuously when they were asked to talk to it, while 64% of the nonstutterers were able to do this and those who could not were "borderline speech defectives". In a study of the eye movements themselves, Strother (1937) found abnormalities of convergence and the presence of considerable nystagmus.

9. *Conclusions*

1. There is no evidence that the stutterer is more likely to be left-handed or ambidextrous than the nonstutterer.

2. The phi-test and intracarotid sodium amytal tests have yielded results suggesting that the stutterer may have incomplete cerebral dominance or bilateral representation of speech.

3. Identical twins do not appear to be more concordant for stuttering than fraternal twins, but the evidence is conflicting.

4. There is no agreement on whether stuttering is more prevalent in families with twins than in those without.

5. A number of studies show that there is more chance of a child developing a stutter if he has relatives who stutter. This relationship cannot be adequately accounted for by the argument that it is the result of association with other stutterers.

6. There is no evidence of any differences in the cardiovascular systems of stutterers and nonstutterers.

7. Two studies report a close relationship between allergic symptoms (including migraine) and stuttering.

8. There is conflicting evidence on whether stutterers have more

carbon dioxide in their blood than nonstutterers and whether the gas is a useful source of treatment. On balance, the evidence is against either being a valid proposition.

9. Stutterers in course of treatment were found to differ from those who had completed treatment in their speech metabolic rate.

10. The appearance of stuttering reported during the administration of a thyroid extract might be accounted for on the grounds that a misdiagnosis was made as to the presence of stuttering. What was observed may have been hurried speech resulting in errors unlike those involved in stuttering.

11. The most promising of the tranquillizing drugs in reducing the frequency of stuttering errors is chlorpromazine, but more research is needed to clarify the position. It is generally reported that all the tranquillizers improve the stutterers' attitude toward their stuttering.

12. There is conflicting evidence on the abnormality of EEG records of stutterers, but over time there is a tendency for more negative than positive results to accrue.

13. There is some evidence that the stutterer could have some minimal disorder of the central nervous system, but this is by no means clearly demonstrated.

14. Stutterers have abnormal patterns of breathing when speaking and probably also in the nonspeaking situation.

15. Grossly discrepant results are reported concerning the motor abilities of people who stutter compared with those who do not. There seems to be a general tendency for the better designed experiments which have used matched samples of subjects to produce negative results.

16. The eye movements of stutterers are possibly atypical of the population in general.

CHAPTER 5

THE PERSONALITY OF STUTTERERS

1. *Introduction*

A great deal of the literature on personality and stuttering has been concerned with identifying what it is which differentiates the stutterer from the nonstutterer, either in terms of specific personality traits or emotional or "neurotic" disturbance. Most of this work has been of the kind in which a test or battery of tests is given in the hope that the stutterers will be shown to be more neurotic, or more introverted (or whatever may be the private belief of the researcher), than a similar group of nonstutterers. This type of thinking is certainly one of the factors responsible for the mass of experiments yielding inconclusive or contradictory results.

In the following pages an attempt will be made to show how the idea of psychological causation for stuttering developed, and this will be followed by some examples of the types of hypothesis and resulting research carried out during this century.

Around the middle of the nineteenth century the search began for psychological causation for speech impediments as an alternative to the assumption that the disorder resulted from some anatomical deformity or physiological malfunctioning. Few would argue that this was an undesirable shift in emphasis. The belief that stuttering arose out of anatomical defects had, for example, led surgeons like Dieffenbach (1841) to cut a transverse wedge out of the tongue and Itard (1817) to use surgical means to "raise" the tongue, while many others had been led to cut out the frenum of the tongue.

Physiological concepts of stuttering did not lead to irreversible surgical procedures but rather to "exercises" and relaxation. Alexander Melville Bell (1853), for example, suggested that loud whispering would be efficacious, while Hagemann (1845) had the stutterer concentrate on keeping the tongue far back on the palate. Still others focused attention on the "spasm" of the stutterer. So interested did people become in this symptom that even today such descriptive names for the speech disorder as labiochorea, spasmophemia, and dysarthria syllabaris spasmodica are used (Bluemel, 1957). On the other hand, relaxation as a therapeutic device was advocated by many specialists (e.g. Hausdoerfer, 1898; Appelt, 1911) and this still plays an important part in many of the treatments of stuttering today.

General interest in the psychological causation of the speech disorder started when Thorné (see Bluemel, 1957) expressed the opinion that stuttering was induced by certain emotions which led to respiratory disturbances, while at the same time still maintaining that the fundamental cause of the defect was an abnormal working of the central nervous system. Thorné thought that there were two groups of psychic conditions which brought about the abnormal speech, one of which consisted of embarrassment, uneasiness, and lack of confidence, while the other was an excessive rapidity of thought with the consequent endeavour to produce the speech with corresponding but disorganizing rapidity.

2. *Stuttering as a Neurotic Manifestation*

Implicit in many theories about the psychological causation in those early years was that stuttering was not a normal but a maladaptive or "neurotic" response.

This became explicit at the beginning of the twentieth century, when certain persons, notably Ssikorski (1894) described stuttering as a psychoneurosis. He believed that the condition was based on a nervous debility of the speech mechanism (thus still retaining the physiological concept) but that each paroxysm was induced by such psychic stimuli as intense eagerness to speak, dread of speaking or too violent innervation when communicating matters which seem of importance to the sufferer.

The supposition that stuttering is a manifestation of an underlying neurotic disorder is still very widely held today. From leading experts in the field we get such statements as

> The neurotic basis of stammering was first noted in the analysis of stammerers in 1913 and 1914 . . . as a result of these investigations, it was finally concluded that stammering is not a speech defect but consists essentially of a persistence into adult life of infantile nursing activities. It could be shown that stammering is one of the severest forms of psychoneurosis, and not merely a tic, an obsession, an auditory amnesis, a spasm of coordination . . . [Coriat, 1943.]

Again, in 1954 Sheehan stated that ". . . stammering . . . is one of the neurotic reactions of a neurotic age". Bluemel is one of the few people who has made some attempt to define what is meant by the term "neurotic"; for him it is a "nervous illness marked by disorganization of bodily functions. The disorganization occurs as a result of stress; and the stress may be either sustained, or sudden and acute" (p. 70).

Probably the best known study in this area is Bender's "The stuttering personality" (1942). Bender gave the Bernreuter Personality Inventory to 249 male college stutterers and a control group of nonstutterers. He reports that, using the six Bernreuter measures, stutterers have a greater neurotic tendency, are more introverted, less dominant, less confident and less sociable. There are, however, at least two criticisms that can be made of this study. First, the distributions on almost all six measures are markedly skewed and hence the parametric statistic employed was not appropriate. Second, there is a substantial correlation between some of the Bernreuter measures, for example 0·95 between neuroticism and introversion scores. So much intercorrelation exists in fact that when Flanagan (1935) factor-analysed the four original Bernreuter measures he found that only two independent dimensions, Confidence and Sociability, could be derived from the inventory. Anastasi (1961) points out that "Scoring keys for these two traits were subsequently added to the test, making a total of six available keys. There is, of course, no justification for using all six keys, since such a practice only further compounds the overlap." (p. 497). In spite of the inappropriate use of statistical and measurement procedures the mean scores obtained on the Bernreuter do suggest that there was a considerable difference in the way in which stutterers and nonstutterers completed the inventory, although one might not be prepared to fully endorse Bender's conclusion that stuttering "is definitely associated with personality maladjustment".

Other investigations using the inventory type test include that of Johnson (1932). He gave the Woodworth House Mental Hygiene Inventory to a group of psychoneurotics and a group of stutterers and concluded that the latter's scores were more like those of the normals in the standardization sample than those of neurotics, except that the stutterers reported significantly more problems than did the normals. In another study Spriestersbach (1951) compared groups of stutterers, normals, and male psychotics on a Word Picture Test of

Social Adjustment. In his survey of research on personality, Goodstein (1958) contends that Spriestersbach's results support those of Johnson in showing that stutterers resemble normal males more than the "psychiatric patients". Such statements help to exemplify the confusion that exists on this topic, for no one has suggested that stutterers are psychotic and in any case Johnson's comparison was with a group of neurotics. There is a further reason why these results cannot be compared with Johnson's. In his paper Spriestersbach describes his test and investigation as an "exploratory study" and states that the results can only be discussed in general terms because of imperfections in design such as the groups showing wide variation in age and educational background. Control of such variables could materially affect the results obtained.

Several investigations have been conducted using the Minnesota Multiphasic Personality Inventory (MMPI) to investigate differences in adjustment between stutterers and others, (e.g. Boland, 1952; Dahlstrom and Craven, 1952; Pizzat, 1949; Thomas, 1951; Walnut, 1954). As an example of the type of result obtained, Table 8 sets out the rank scores for each of the four groups used by Walnut. Since nothing below the seventieth percentile rank can be considered to be clinically significant, the scores of all groups are clearly well within normal limits and one would be guarded in one's acceptance of statements such as

> In comparing the pathological groups and the control group in the study the following differences were observed: (a) The stuttering group showed significant differences on the Depression and Paranoid scales . . . and these differences were toward the poor adjustment end of the scale. According to the MMPI manual, this would indicate that in relation to others of comparable experience, the stuttering group has (1) "poor adjustment of the emotional type with a feeling of uselessness and inability to assume normal optimism with regard to the future", and is characterized by (2) "suspiciousness, oversensitivity, and delusions of persecution". [p. 222.]

By far the largest group of studies of the relationship between stuttering and personality has employed projective techniques. Not everyone would agree with Sheehan (1958a) that this is evidence of the increasing sophistication of clinical psychology, the trend being from "psychometric to paper–pencil tests, and finally projective tests. The better recent research has utilized projective techniques, particularly the Rorschach and the Thematic Apperception Test (TAT)" (p. 18). The alternative view might be held that, because of the well-documented invalidity and unreliability of projective tests, trends in the direction of making greater use of these techniques would be a retrograde step.

TABLE 8

Ranks of all four groups according to the clinical scale of the MMPI (Walnut, 1954, p. 221)

	Control group	Stuttering group	Crippled group	Cleft palate group
Hypochondriasis	49	42	49	51
Depression	51	53	52	54
Hysteria	53	48	53	52
Psychopathic deviation	55	45	52	49
Interest	50	55	49	55
Paranoia	50	54	49	51
Psychasthenia	52	52	49	51
Schizophrenic	56	49	53	50
Hypomania	58	52	52	52

However, in reviewing the literature on projective studies of stuttering Sheehan warns that one must be cautious in accepting authors' interpretations of their statistical results. He cites the study by Krugman (1946) in which the results were interpreted as showing that the child stutterers manifested the obsessive-compulsive type of personality trait but that the statistical results were in direct contradiction to this interpretation. That confusion such as this is common is further exemplified by the study of Meltzer (1944) who used the Rorschach to study the differences in responses of both stuttering and normal speaking children, and found significant differences on W, Z and $F+$ measures. However, Meltzer also proceeds to interpret scores for individuals *within* the stuttering group, even though their mean scores do not differ from those of the control group, and from such an analysis concludes that "Within the stuttering group are found children whose M's indicate not only creative ability but a tendency to fantasy and withdrawal." Similarly, on the basis of a difference significant at the 25% level, Meltzer states that "It seems safe to say that the stuttering children have a greater tendency towards morbidity and sterotypy in thought and action than does the control group" (p. 51).

These studies of Krugman and Meltzer which conclude that the stuttering child is neurotic in terms of the most ephemeral evidence are directly contradicted by Wilson (1951) and Christensen (1952). These latter investigators used the child's normal speaking sibling as the control and interpreted their Rorschach and TAT scores as suggesting that there was no real difference in neuroticism or maladjustment between the two groups, although Wilson did report that the stutterers were more aggressive and had more "inverted hostility".

Similar contradictions in results of studies using projective tests have been found with adults. For instance, Haney (1950) and Pitrelli (1948) both thought that the stutterers' responses on the Rorschach were suggestive of a neurotic disorder but neither used a control group. On the other hand, Richardson (1944) found no significant differences between stutterers and nonstutterers on the TAT and no differences in mean scores on the Rorschach, but did find that the stutterers showed greater variability and that "In proportion of responses on the Rorschach Test, the only significant difference found was in the instance where there were no M (movement) and C (colour) responses. The stutterers tended not to recognise their inner life and not to respond impulsively to their outer environment" (p. 37).

Another projective test that has received the attention of research workers is the Rosenzweig Picture Frustration Test. Madison and Norman (1952) used this test to examine Abbott's (1947) contention that stutterers may be reluctant to discard their secondary symptoms during treatment. The argument involved was that repressed hostility toward the listener produces unconscious guilt feelings, and the stutterers' symptoms fulfil the need of the stutterer for self-punishment as an atonement for this hostility. The authors compared the responses of 25 stutterers with Rosenzweig's normative data and found the results supported the psychoanalytic notion that stuttering is compulsive in nature with "anal-sadistic tendencies resulting in a turning inwards of aggression". No mention is made in this study as to the source of interpretation of responses, and the possibility of contamination effects might account for Quarrington's (1953) inability to replicate these findings.

It is by no means the rule in studies using projective tests to ensure that the judges who carry out the assessment of protocols are unaware of the purpose of the study as well as which protocol belongs to which experimental group. As with many other studies mentioned, both Madison and Norman and Quarrington used the normative test data and not a matched control group.

One point of particular interest in the Madison and Norman experiment was the separate analysis of responses of male and female stutterers and of the group as a whole. For example, while the male, female and total stutterer group results were significant ($p < 0.001$) in indicating more intropunitive responses when compared with the normative data, only the male and total groups were significantly different ($p < 0.05$) in terms of lessened extrapunitive tendency. Again, only the females were significantly higher on Need–Persistence ($p < 0.05$). Such observations as these suggest the operation of factors accounting for the many discrepant results obtained since, in this type of research, groups of mixed sex are most often used. Even if this were not the case it is of some importance to establish whether sex differences such as those indicated are present when the main aim of the research is to determine whether stutterers are more neurotic than nonstutterers. Anastasi (1958) has stressed that the normative data of personality tests indicates that women tend to obtain more neurotic or maladjusted scores than men and in view of this it is surprising that sometimes research workers do not take this into account.

The most striking aspect concerning this group of studies is the inconclusive results. Whether this is due to contamination effects, lack of controls, badly matched samples or incorrect interpretation of results is of importance when future studies are being considered, and it must be hoped that due consideration will be given to the importance of these factors in future research design.

3. *General Personality Characteristics of the Stutterer*

There have been many studies purporting to investigate whether or not stutterers are characterized by a particular cluster of traits which distinguishes them from the nonstutterer, but in fact the main emphasis has been upon examination for presence or absence of neurotic traits. As will be appreciated, some of the studies reported in the last section indicate that information on other types of personality characteristic is to be found and a few studies are specially designed with this aim in mind.

For example, there is Bender's (1942) reported finding that 249 male college stutterers were significantly less confident and less sociable than 249 male college nonstutterers. As mentioned previously, Flanagan found that two factors (Confidence and Sociability) could be substituted for Bernreuter's original four and this suggests that there is little justification in discussing results based upon the original trait labels.

Two investigators have used the Guildford Inventory of Factors STDCR with the usual pattern of conflicting results (Richardson, 1944; Shames, 1949). For example, Richardson found her stutterers to be "more socially introverted, more depressed and less happy-go-lucky than the nonstutterers" (p. 37), while Shames' could not be said to differ in these respects. Yet, as with so many studies, this was not a complete replication of Richardson's experiment, because Shames did not employ a control group but rather compared his stutterers' scores with the test norms.

One cannot escape the observation that the mass of reported studies on the personality of stutterers is heavily weighted with negative findings; it seems much easier to show in what ways the stutterer does *not* differ from the nonstutterer than ways in which he does. He does not appear to differ from the nonstutterer in his sense of humour (Staats, 1955), responses on the Kent–Rosanoff Word Association Test (Font, 1955), obsessive-compulsive reactions (Bloodstein and Schreiber, 1957), achievement motivation (Goodstein *et al.*, 1955) or in aggression and orality (Lowinger, 1952).

Just as there is no real evidence to justify the conclusion that stuttering is related to maladjustment, so the search for a consistent personality profile of the stutterer seems to have failed. Where differences have been found they have often failed to be successfully cross-validated; inadequate statistical procedures have been used; they have lacked proper controls; or been subject to experimenter bias. Also, of the few studies which have yielded seemingly reliable differences, positive results are rarer than negative. It could well be argued that if the stutterer has a unique personality pattern this should have been abundantly apparent by this time.

4. *Investigations of Specific Personality Variables*

Over the years there has been an increasing tendency to concentrate upon more specific personality variables and to abandon the attempt to try to isolate a "general stuttering personality" profile. The specific personality variables mainly studied have been "rigidity", "level of aspiration", "self concept", "anxiety", and "hostility".

It was Eisenson (1937) who first reported that stutterers show more perseveration than nonstutterers, and Kapos and Fattu (1957) who found there to be significantly more behavioural rigidity in severely speech-handicapped children than in normal speaking children. Kapos and Standlee (1958) followed this up by an investigation of whether or not there was any carry-over of the perseveration demonstrated by stutterers in their fixed speech patterns to behavioural rigidity; but they were unable to find evidence for this in their group of stutterers and nonstutterers. This research is discussed in more detail in Chapter 3.

One area of investigation in which research has fairly consistently demonstrated some difference between stutterers and normal speakers is in level of aspiration; the evidence suggests that stutterers underestimate their abilities. The first studies of this variable were not encouraging, for example Sheehan and Zelen (1951) failed to find differences at a significant level between 20 stutterers and 20 nonstutterers in discrepancy scores obtained on the Rotter level of aspiration board, but they did note that the stutterers obtained somewhat lower scores than the nonstutterers.

In a later study (1955), however, these authors carried out an investigation using 40 stutterers and 60 matched controls and this time the stutterers did show a significantly lower discrepancy between aim and accomplishment $(p < 0.05)$ and a significantly higher success rate $(p < 0.02)$. An additional finding of interest was that whereas there were no sex differences in scores obtained by the controls, the female stutterers scored significantly lower than the male stutterers $(p < 0.01)$. The authors show understandable interest in this finding, pointing out that one of the many mysteries of stuttering is the sex ratio, the disorder being three to four times more common in men than in women.

Another study using level of aspiration discrepancy scores as a discriminator between stutterers and nonstutterers was carried out by Mast (1951). He did not analyse male and female differences on these scores but he reported that stutterers had significantly lower scores and interpreted this as indicating that their defences against failure were more exaggerated than in the case of nonstutterers.

It seems, therefore, that there is no consistent evidence to justify the conclusion that stutterers are particularly rigid in their behaviour when this is defined as an inability to change from one sequence of responses to another. But the position is slightly clearer when dealing with level of aspiration. All the experiments have yielded results tending to suggest that the stutterer has less discrepancy between the score he predicts he will make on a test and the one he actually achieves.

5. *The Self Concept*

The term "self concept", as commonly used, refers to the "self as the individual who is known to himself" (English and English, 1958). It is obviously difficult to measure this self concept, but in recent years attempts have been made to do this in a systematic way. One of the chief exponents of the importance of the self concept is Rogers (1951) who based much of his work upon the classic study of Raimy (1948). Raimy postulated three basic principles with respect to the self concept: (i) the self concept is a learned perceptual system which functions as an object in the perceptual field; (ii) the self concept not only influences behaviour but is itself altered and restructured by behaviour and unsatisfied needs; (iii) it may have little or no relation to external reality.

Very similar concepts have played a dominant role in other theories, in particular that of Snygg and Combs (1949). Their basic postulate is that "all behaviour without exception, is completely determined by and pertinent to the phenomenal field of the organism". In all such theories an individual's frame of reference is his Not-Self or Environment and his Phenomenal Self. When any inconsistency arises the individual acts in such a way as to regain consistency. What may appear as irrational behaviour to the observer is held to be understandable if one were only aware of the existing inconsistency between the self concepts and the perceptions of external reality.

The Zeitgeist which is prevalent in general psychology has been reflected in the literature on stuttering and there has been increasing emphasis on the importance of the self-concept of the stutterer. As long ago as 1945 Van Riper outlined thirteen steps a stutterer could take to acclimatize himself gradually to more difficult situations and although one goal was the elimination of the stutter another was advocated to enable the stutterer to accept his speech defect as part of his true self. Similarly Shearer (1961) suggests that relapses occur if the stutterer ceases to perceive himself as one who stutters and thus fails to monitor his speech in such a way as to be aware of mild blocks and subtle environmental cues which tend to elicit stuttering. Shearer in fact described a therapy programme much of which is "devoted to reconciling the two conflicting self-concepts, the horrible stuttering self and the free-speaking normal self". A similar therapeutic approach has also been advocated by Bryngelson *et al.* (1950) as well as by Johnson (1946).

Not only does the concept of the self play an important part in much contemporary speech therapy but it is also held by Sheehan (1954) that a considerable part of the stutterers' resistance to cure may be explained in terms of a dichotomized self concept. This notion is based on the observation that stutterers tend to leave therapy just when the therapist believes that improvement is taking place, and all who deal with stutterers are aware that many have tried every available treatment without apparent improvement. Sheehan finds support for his idea by pointing out that the stutterer can become very anxious when he is asked such questions as "if your stuttering suddenly disappeared, what difference would it make in your life" (p. 480). He suggests that such anxiety arises because the stutterer uses his defect as an excuse for all his shortcomings, or possibly because "he may have lived with his stuttering so long that functioning without it involves too radical a change in self-concept to be radically assimilated" (p. 480). If this is so then Sheehan suggests that just as in the early stages of treatment "the stutterer needs to accept himself as a stutterer, so in the final stages he must learn to accept himself as a normal speaker" (p. 480). By accepting the latter he then gives up the secondary gains which have led him to retain his speech defect and also "acquires a radically different self concept".

The self concept is clearly given prominence in several therapeutic programmes and the relationship between this factor and the speech disorder is of considerable interest, but its value depends upon the discovery of satisfactory methods for its assessment so that the changes occurring during treatment can be studied and any hypothesized relationships examined.

There have been some attempts to measure the self concepts of stutterers and the following three to be mentioned have been aimed at examining whether the self concepts of stutterers differ from those of nonstutterers. Both Fiedler and Wepman (1951) and Wallen (1959) used Stephenson's Q-technique (1950). This technique is a method for quantifying the relationship between certain concepts of a person and comparing these relationships with those of other subjects. In these two experiments the technique was employed to assess the degree to which different types of people varied in their perceptions of themselves and others. Fiedler and Wepman employed 76 statements descriptive of personality traits and found that, in terms of these, the stutterers' self concept did not differ from that of non-stutterers. Wallen approached the matter in a slightly different way. He used 100 self-referent statements made by stutterers which were then sorted into six personality trait areas; these being (i) self-acceptance, (ii) independence, (iii) self-rejection, (iv) dependence, (v) lack of emotional control and (vi) withdrawal. These 100 statements were sorted by the stutterers and nonstutterers in terms of "how I think I really am", "how I would like to be" and "how I think others see me". The results showed the stutterers to be significantly lower on self-acceptance and independence $(p < 0 \cdot 001)$, and significantly higher on self-rejection and lack of emotional control $(p < 0 \cdot 001)$. The stutterers also exhibited a significantly lower congruence between the actual self/ideal-self relationship. This approach was possibly more successful in isolating differences between the two groups since it did not try to identify an overall similarity in self concept profile and the statements had been selected as being directly relevant. It would have been interesting had the concept "how I think stutterers are" been given to the nonstutterers and the results compared with the stutterers' actual performance.

Wylie (1961) has criticized the Q-sort on several grounds including that of there being too little information on the reliability of the scores so derived and in terms of their validity as measures of the self. The present authors would concur with Vernon (1964) in recognizing that all Wylie's criticisms should be given serious attention but that the instrument is proving useful in studies of therapeutic change and personality research.

Lower self-acceptance scores for stutterers (and prisoners) than for college student nonstutterers have been reported by Berger (1952). He constructed his own inventory which had matched-half reliabilities for various subgroups of $0 \cdot 75$. The questionnaire has not been published so that one is not able to assess the possible effects of the tendencies some subjects have to accept more statements as applicable to themselves than others (acquiescence) or to be more extreme in

their responses irrespective of the content of the item (extreme-
ness).

Yet another technique was used by Zelen *et al.* (1954). This is
called the Who-Are-You or W-A-Y technique. Its approach is
more direct in that the person is asked the question "Who are you?"
and the responses to this question are sorted into eleven categories.
The overall *F*-ratio calculated between responses of a group of
stutterers and a group of nonstutterers on this measure was significant at the 5% level, stutterers giving significantly more responses
that were classified under positive affect and group membership, and
significantly fewer responses classified under uniqueness of respon-
dent, age and sex.

It is not possible to compare this study with that of Fiedler and
Wepman in any meaningful way because both the method of
measurement and procedure are so totally different. It is also rather
an unsatisfactory study on several counts. One is told that the samples
consisted of 30 stutterers and 160 nonstutterers but that the latter
had been used in previous studies. It seems rather unlikely that these
groups were adequately matched on what might be considered
relevant variables, nor is it possible to assess the statistical results
since no figures whatever are published except the probability levels.
Perhaps the most difficult thing to accept is the seemingly arbitrary
nature of the interpretations. For instance, the authors state that the
finding that stutterers had more positive feelings about themselves

> can be interpreted in either of two ways; (1) that stutterers tend to over-
> compensate for their feelings of inferiority and so protect themselves with a
> halo of positive feeling; (2) more fundamentally perhaps, that these particular
> stutterers, having decided to help themselves through psychotherapy, had
> resolved a major conflict in their phenomenal field and thus had more
> positive feelings about themselves.

In accounting for the lower number of responses in the Unit, Age
and Sex categories, the authors state that "this may be interpreted
as being a function of the stutterer's lessened concern with a census-
type perceptual orientation and having instead a heightened orientation to his problems" (p. 71).

In another study, Sheehan and Martyn (1966) asked stutterers and
"recovered stutterers" specific questions about their "self concept"
and report that the incorporation of stuttering into the self concept
is related to the probability of spontaneous recovery ($p < 0.001$).
They go on to say that "whether stuttering persists is . . . largely a
function of how the stutterer views himself and how he feels about

himself in relation to others" (p. 130). The degree of confidence which can be attached to this statement, however, must depend upon the reliance which can be placed upon a person's report of the kind of person they thought or remembered themselves to be anything up to 40 years ago.

Another study which has been concerned with the self concept of the stutterer is that of Fransella (1965a) in which the repertory grid and a form of semantic differential were used. Repertory grid technique is a method devised by Kelly (1955) to measure the basic units

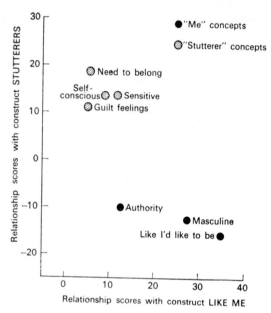

FIG. 9. Mean relationship scores of constructs with the constructs "stutterers" and "like me" on a repertory grid (Fransella, 1965a).

in his Personal Construct Theory. In this theory the individual is again the centre of attention and it is held that his behaviour becomes understandable if one knows the constructs he uses to interpret the events in his environment. To Kelly the self concept is but one of the yardsticks man uses to enable him to control and predict events. The semantic differential, as described by Osgood *et al.* (1957), and the repertory grid have many points in common but the latter is a more indirect method of measurement.

Fransella was concerned to investigate whether the stutterer attached the same meaning to the concept "Stutterer" as he did to his concept of "Me", rather than to see whether the stutterer differed in his self concept from the nonstutterer. Figure 9 shows the constructs used plotted according to their mean correlation (squared) with the constructs "Like Me" and "Like Stutterers", on the repertory grid. A statistical analysis of the construct relationships derived from the repertory grid, and of the clustering on the semantic differential, showed that on both measures the "Self" concepts

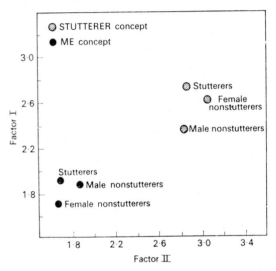

FIG. 10. Factor scores of concepts "stutterers" and "me" for groups of stutterers and nonstutterers on the Speech Correction Semantic Differential (a constant of 2·0 has been added) (Fransella, 1965a).

differed significantly from the "Stutterer" concepts ($p < 0.005$ on the repertory grid and < 0.001 on the semantic differential). Fransella suggested that the stutterer does not necessarily have a dual self concept but, more probably, that he has one constellation of concepts which are used to describe himself, and another to describe stutterers. This is to say he accepts that he stutters but not that he is like other stutterers as a person; in other words, he is in some way unique.

It is perhaps of interest to note that when male and female nonstutterers rated the same concepts on the semantic differential their ratings did not differ significantly from those of the stutterers. Figure 10 shows how closely the groups agree in the meaning they ascribe to the concepts "Me" and "Stutterers".

The evidence seems to suggest that being a stutterer forms part of the stutterer's self concept when direct questions are asked but does not necessarily do so when measurement is more indirect.

6. *Anxiety and Hostility*

Several studies have been directly concerned with anxiety and its relation to stuttering but these have been mainly concerned with situations or words which are thought to influence the stutterer's "level of anxiety". It is surprising that there have been relatively few investigations of whether the stutterer has or does not have a higher level of anxiety in general than the nonstutterer. Two studies have reported results indicating that this group is characterized by significantly higher levels of general anxiety as measured by two inventories (Boland, 1952) and by a projective test (Santostefano, 1960). This latter assumed the stutterer to be under constant stress because of the negative evaluations made of him by both himself and his environment. This stress was assumed to produce "predominant and enduring states of anxiety and hostility". It was therefore hypothesized that stutterers would gain higher anxiety and hostility scores than nonstutterers on the Rorschach test. An additional hypothesis put forward was that such anxiety and hostility would have a disruptive effect when the stutterer was subjected to stress in a laboratory situation.

Both hypotheses were supported by the results of the personality test and by experiment and thus confirming the common observation that the stutterer appears to have a generally higher level of anxiety than the nonstutterer, in addition to having increased anxiety in specific situations and to specific words. However, other results were obtained when a physiological measure of anxiety was used. While studying the relationship between adaptation and anxiety in stutterers and nonstutterers Karmen (1964) found no difference in anxiety level between stutterers and nonstutterers. One explanation of these discrepant findings might be that both Boland and Santostefano had selected stutterers whose speech defect was moderately severe, and Karmen (1964) reports that her subgroup of "moderate" stutterers had significantly higher anxiety scores than either the "high" or "low" stutterers.

7. Stutterer Subgroups

The question of whether research workers are justified in subsuming all people who have a certain defect of speech under the heading of "stutterers" has already been discussed. On reading the literature summarized in each of the chapters of this book it becomes apparent that many isolated attempts are being made to subdivide this all-embracing category.

In the field of personality and stuttering one of the most interesting attempts at subdivision is that of Douglass and Quarrington (1952). They have distinguished between "interiorized" and "exteriorized" stuttering, the former being characterized by constant vigilance to avoid stuttering, while the latter is characterized by overt speech abnormality, the main goal being to communicate and any avoidance devices used are to facilitate speech.

These authors are of the opinion that the two groups of stutterers differ in terms of the behaviour and devices they use, in personality and self-concepts, in social mobility, and in terms of stuttering development. The interiorized stutterer tends to be sensitive, submissive and retiring, and is very concerned about any spasm he sees or hears himself make. The exteriorized stutterer, on the other hand, assumes that he is accepted in society, is aggressive, regards authorities as threatening and never believes he really looked or sounded as abnormal as he can be shown to be. A further subdivision proposed is that stuttering can be either vocalized or nonvocalized. Vocalized stuttering is seen as an audibly perceived phenomenon in which repetition or prolongation of sounds predominate, while nonvocalized stuttering is a visually perceived phenomenon characterized by blocking or suspension of speech.

Quarrington and Douglass (1960) conducted an experiment which set out to test the hypothesis that, of the two subgroups of exteriorized stuttering, the nonvocalized stutterer would have a stronger drive to avoid allowing the disorder to become audible. The experiment consisted of having a group of vocalized and a group of nonvocalized stutterers read a different passage of prose under two conditions. In one condition the subject knew that he could be heard, while in the other he was given the impression that his reading would not be heard. It was predicted that the nonvocalized stutterer would show a greater reduction in audible stuttering than the vocalized stutterer under the condition of not being heard as this would be less anxiety-provoking for him. The results of this experiment were as predicted and the authors suggest that this implies that the two groups of stutterers should be given somewhat different types of treatment.

Doust (1956) also divided his stutterers into interiorized, exteriorized nonvocal and exteriorized vocal, when investigating responses to the stress of breath holding. As can be seen in Table 9 there is

TABLE 9

Stress scores in stutterers, normals and neurotics (Doust, 1956)

Type of stuttering	N	Mean oximetric stress response score	S.D.
Exteriorized nonvocal	14	+34·714	12·969
Exteriorized vocal	18	+35·000	18·471
Interiorized	13	+38·200	13·200
Cluttering	1	+35·000	—
Dyslalia	1	+33·000	—
Fluent controls	112	+14·625	10·741
Fluent neurotics	64	− 0·859	11·447

no difference in the responses made by these subgroups; all over-respond. The marked difference between the stutterers' stress scores and those of the fluent controls and neurotics leads Doust to conclude that this "provides further evidence that stutterers are not neurotics" (p. 33).

8. *Test Scores as Prognostic Indicators*

It is of considerable importance when considering the treatment of any complaint to be able to assess the probability and degree of improvement. As yet there is little in the literature on stuttering to give the therapist much guide as to what features may be regarded as good or bad prognostic indicators. One study with this important consideration in mind was conducted by Sheehan et al. (1954), who set out to test the validity of the Rorschach Prognostic Rating Scale (Klopfer *et al.*, 1951) by administering it to a population of 35 stutterers. They compared the scores of those judged most improved and those judged least improved by their therapists, and also compared those who stayed in therapy with those who dropped out. Separate ratings were made of psychotherapeutic and speech improvements. The finding that the scale discriminated significantly between "improvers" and "nonimprovers" cannot, unfortunately, be accepted unequivocally as it would appear that the same people carried out the administration and scoring of the Rorschach protocols as well as the ratings and the treatment. This would inevitably involve considerable contamination of results, the therapist being aware of those individuals having high or low prognosis scores. Similarly, when making pre- and post-therapy comparisons each individual would have all the available information. The authors conclude that the scale is successful in predicting psychological change but no improvement in speech.

Shames (1952) investigated prognosis in therapy for stutterers, using the Guildford–Martin Inventory of Factors STDCR and the Rorschach test for this purpose. He also obtained measures of speech adequacy from pre- and post-recordings of samples of speech and ratings of the amount of avoidance observed in social situations. He points out that the same people did *not* make the speech and social avoidance measures. He then calculated the chi-squares between each of these four evaluations of speech therapy and each of forty variables that might be related to prognosis. From all these statistics only eleven were significant and Shames points out that one would expect sixteen to be significant at the 10% level by chance alone. He argues that the study had value in suggesting certain refinements in the design of this type of research and also in demonstrating that research on prognosis and evaluation of therapy can be carried out without disturbing the clinical situation.

In a more recent study, Lanyon (1966) assessed the relationship between improvement in stuttering therapy and certain measures on the MMPI, the latter having been previously shown to be related to change in psychotherapy (Barron, 1953; Marks and Seeman, 1963; Dahlstrom and Welsh, 1960). Two of the four MMPI variables were significant in the predicted direction, although the correlations concerned were not high (0·46 and −0·38) and therefore only tentative comments are made about the findings. In particular it was suggested that the person who improves after stuttering therapy tends to be similar to those improving following psychotherapy in that they are both adaptable and resourceful. Those benefiting from stuttering therapy also may not be basically deviant in terms of personality and thinking patterns. Lanyon concludes by saying that further research into what personality factors may be favourable to improvement in stuttering therapy is indicated.

9. *Conclusions*

1. There is no evidence to suggest that the stutterer has a particular type of personality or group of traits that differentiates him from the nonstutterer.

2. No evidence exists that stutterers find it more difficult to change over from one set of response patterns to another than do nonstutterers.

3. Stutterers have been shown to have significantly less discrepancy on a test between what they aim at and what they accomplish than do nonstutterers.

4. The evidence on the self concept of stutterers is conflicting, but it seems as if they may be less ready to accept themselves as they are. They may also perceive stutterers as a group as having certain personality characteristics that they do not ascribe to themselves.

5. Stutterers appear to have a higher general level of anxiety than nonstutterers but there is too little evidence to be certain of this. There may also be differences in anxiety level between certain subgroups of stutterers.

6. At a descriptive level interiorized stutterers are distinguished from exteriorized stutterers. There is support for the idea that stutterers in the latter category who show more blocks than overt stutterers are more highly motivated to avoid stuttering than vocalized stutterers.

7. There is as yet no usable method for predicting which individual stutterer will improve in treatment.

8. There is little unequivocal evidence that stutterers as a group are more neurotic or maladjusted than nonstutterers.

9. Studies investigating the personality of stutterers are characterized by interpretations that are at variance with the statistical findings; contamination effects resulting from the person who conducts the experiment also being the one who scores the projective

tests or assesses outcome of treatment; lack of adequate control groups; inappropriate or inadequate statistical treatment. There has also been hardly any attempt to take into account that female stutterers may not have similar personality traits to male stutterers or that they may be more neurotic.

CHAPTER 6

EXPERIMENTAL INVESTIGATIONS OF THREE BASIC PHENOMENA OF STUTTERING

A. THE CONSISTENCY AND EXPECTANCY EFFECTS

1. *Description*

The term "consistency effect" was first used by Johnson and Knott (1937) to describe the observation that stutterers tend to stutter on the same words when reading the same passage several times. This notion has been extended by some investigators (e.g. Berwick, 1955; Brown, 1945; Connett, 1955; Fierman, 1955) to cover a consistent tendency to stutter in the presence of the same environmental cues or stimuli.

Johnson and Knott (1937) reported that about 60–70% of stutterings occurred on the same words and no findings have been reported since then which unequivocally contradict this. It seems that individual stutterers not only find certain words or sounds always more difficult than others but that they tend also to respond consistently even when the stimulus situation is varied. Shulman (1955) compared the consistency of stuttering when a passage of prose was read five times in the presence of one person, with a situation in which the number of people present increased by one with each successive reading and she found differences in consistency scores only with respect to the first and second reading.

Not only is this effect characteristic of the speech behaviour of almost all stutterers but it seems also to be highly related to severity of stuttering. Shulman (1955) reports a correlation between consistency and severity of 0·66, while Tate and Cullinan (1962) found such correlations for five consistency measures to range from 0·67 to 0·93.

126

2. *Scoring*

Tate and Cullinan (1962) consider that two points have to be taken into account when assessing the "consistency" performance of individuals: (i) how many of the repeated word-stutterings can be expected to occur by chance alone, and (ii) how can the statistical significance of the difference between the amount of observed and expected consistency be assessed.

The most usual way of measuring consistency is to calculate the percentage of words stuttered during any one reading which were also stuttered in a previous reading. It could be argued that the correlation of $0 \cdot 66$ between this measure and severity of stuttering (Shulman, 1955) was due to the fact that the more stuttering which occurs, the more likelihood there is of repeated stutterings on the same word. But Tate and Cullinan found that high correlations with severity were apparent even when the measures they were using made allowance for such chance factors. They investigated five measures of consistency and concluded that the "percentage" measure was "clearly unsatisfactory". Three of the other measures correlated very highly together and, with two of these, tests of significance can be used (the maximum difference and normal deviate scores). Of these scores they consider the normal deviate score the more flexible and the easier to compute. This index is expressed in the formula

$$z = \frac{|O_o - E_o| - \frac{1}{2}}{\sqrt{E_o (N - E_o)/N}}$$

where O_o is the observed number of nonstuttered words and E_o the expected number. Since this is a standard score and thus normally distributed (providing E_o or $N - E_o$, whichever is the smaller, is about 5 or more), the normal probability scale can be directly applied.

3. *Expectancy and Adaptation*

As has already been pointed out, the consistency effect seems to be a characteristic found in the speech of nearly all stutterers, and it is Bloodstein's view (1960a) that the stutterers' blocks are "precipitated by certain evaluations or preconceptions which the stutterer entertains about these points in the speech sequence".

That the stutterer *knows* that he is going to stutter on a word is apparent from the literature on expectancy which has been clearly summarized by Wischner (1952). The usual procedure for obtaining an estimate of expectancy is to ask the stutterer to indicate, during silent reading, each word on which he considers he would experience difficulty if he were to read aloud.

The degree of accuracy with which the stutterer is able to predict his stutterings is quite considerable. In Knott, Johnson and Webster's (1937) group, 94–96% of the anticipated words were stuttered on as opposed to only 0·4–3% of those not anticipated. When the anticipated "difficult" words were deleted 98% of the stuttering was eliminated (Johnson and Sinn, 1937).

Van Riper (1936) was able to predict words on which the stutterers would expect difficulty by the Inspiration–Expiration duration ratio occurring immediately after the word was shown to the subject. Other physiological correlates of the expectancy phenomenon, such as change in pulse rate and neck rigidity, have been observed by many people and are reported in Van Riper and Milisen (1939). Some children, however, are not able to say in advance that they are going to stutter on a certain word before they do, yet these same children show consistency of stuttering in the reading situation. It had indeed been pointed out (Johnson and Sinn, 1937; Johnson and Solomon, 1937) that anticipation need not necessarily be a conscious process. One explanation of this could be that *if* stuttering is a conditioned response, then the anticipation could be the conscious awareness of the conditioned response already established. This is perhaps a more useful way of thinking about the phenomenon than talking about "subliminal" anticipation, such as Bloodstein infers must exist simply because the consistency effect exists.

Bloodstein (1960a) has supplied some very interesting evidence which suggests that children between the ages of 3 and 6, who some might call "primary stutterers", also stutter on an average on 77·1% of the same words in a sentence dictated to them twice. He is of the opinion that this evidence alone throws doubt on the validity of any theory which attempts to differentiate between simple repetitions and blockings. He prefers to see stuttering as the steady development of anticipatory struggle responses.

4. *Word Analysis*

It seems clear that stutterers can predict words on which they will stutter so that the question arises as to the basis on which the prediction is made. Brown (1945) has suggested that the stutterer evaluates the words that he is going to speak and, according to his evaluation, will expect to stutter more or less. Since the stutterer always uses the same criteria to assess the degree of difficulty of the words, he will exhibit consistency of stuttering on those words. Brown isolated four criteria that the stutterer seems to use in evaluating his words and if words are weighted in terms of these criteria prior to reading, it is possible to predict the extent to which they will be likely to elicit stuttering.

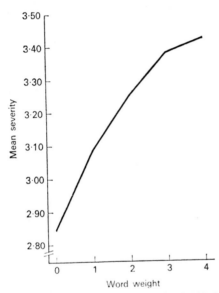

Fig. 11. Mean severity of stuttering on words classified according to Brown's word weights (redrawn from Trotter, 1956).

Brown's factors for word weighting are:

(i) words that begin with sounds that were shown by Johnson and Brown (1935) to cause more than $9 \cdot 7\%$ of stuttering;

(ii) words that are adjectives, nouns, adverbs or verbs;

(iii) words that come first, second or third in the sentence;

(iv) words that have five or more letters.

Oxtoby (1955) supported Brown's findings by reporting that the number of times a word was stuttered was proportional to the number of the above characteristics it possessed. It has also been found (Trotter, 1956) that the actual *severity* of stuttering on a word is related to its weighting on the above factors as shown in Fig. 11.

A considerable amount of work has been done in recent years on trying to define more clearly the factors underlying the effectiveness of Brown's word-weighting criteria, and each will be dealt with in turn.

(a) Initial sounds

In 1935 Johnson and Brown stated that it was possible to rank the initial sounds of words in order of speaking difficulty, some consonants being more difficult for stutterers than others and, in particular, consonants in general being more likely to cause stuttering than vowels. In this early study no attempt was made to take into account the other three factors suggested by Brown which might have been likely to interact with the consonant/vowel factor. Similarly, Hahn (1942) did not control for these factors when confirming Johnson and Brown's finding that vowels are easier for stutterers than consonants.

More recently, Quarrington et al. (1962) investigated the interrelationship between initial letter or sound, grammatical form and word position in the sentence. They argued that since Hejna (1955) had failed to find any difference between consonants in the amount of stuttering elicited, and since there was a very high level of intersubject variability in the difficulty experienced with the different sounds, it might be that one of Brown's criteria has no validity.

Equating words for length and frequency of usage, they constructed 64 sentences which included experimental words (a) placed in the initial or terminal position, (b) having initial letter (consonant) of high or low stuttering frequency and (c) belonging to the grammatical categories nouns, adjectives, adverbs and verbs. In Figure 12 it will be seen that initial words produced considerably more stuttering than did the terminal words ($p < 0.005$) and that the grammatical form of the words is related to the frequency of stuttering ($p < 0.005$). As for the initial sound of the word, this interacted ($p < 0.025$) with both position and grammatical form of the word but produced no significant effect in its own right. Soderberg (1962) extended this result by finding no significant difference between vowels and two types of consonant. This is certainly contrary to previous results which have been quite clear in showing vowels to be easier than consonants.

Taylor (1966a) inspected Soderberg's test material and suggests that these discrepant results may have been caused by the inadvertent under-representation of difficult consonants and over-representation of easy ones, and by the fact that the different sounds did not appear equally at each position in the phrases of the test lists. Taylor (1966b) used a multiple regression analysis on data elicited from 9 subjects reading a passage of prose three times. She did not examine the differential stuttering frequency within the group of consonants but

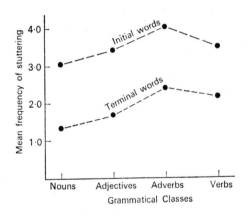

FIG. 12. Frequency of stuttering related to grammatical class of initial and terminal critical words (redrawn from Quarrington *et al.*, 1962).

found that the consonant/vowel difference was highly significant statistically ($p < 0.001$).

The observation of Quarrington *et al.* (1962) that the difficulties in finding significant differences between consonants may be due to high variability between subjects was supported by their finding of a significant Subject by Initial Consonant Phonemes interaction ($p < 0.01$).

Thus, there is substantial evidence from these studies that more stuttering is to be expected on consonants than on vowels, but it still has to be demonstrated that stutterers as a group find some consonants more difficult than others.

(b) Grammatical form

Brown (1937) had found that adjectives, nouns, verbs and adverbs were more likely to elicit stuttering than other parts of speech and Taylor (1966b) obtained a correlation of 0·89 when she ranked Brown's subjects in terms of the difficulty they experienced on the different parts of speech. Figure 12 (Quarrington *et al.*, 1962) also shows that the grammatical form of the words is related to frequency of stuttering ($p < 0·005$), but the order of difficulty is very different. This could be accounted for by the fact that in Brown's study no attempt was made to control for word length or position; certain grammatical forms tend to be placed in certain positions in sentences and to be of different length. When Taylor (1966b) divided the words into "content" (nouns, verbs, adverbs and adjectives) and "function" words, these correlated with stuttering 0·12 ($p < 0·05$), the "content" words producing more stuttering.

All studies report results indicating that some grammatical forms are more difficult for stutterers than others, but there is considerable variability between stutterers.

(c) Position in the phrase or sentence

As already mentioned, Quarrington *et al.* (1962) found that more stuttering occurred on the first than on the last word of a sentence ($p < 0·005$). In a later study he (1965) reported a correlation of $-0·49$ between frequency of stuttering and word position, indicating that the earlier a word came in the sentence the more likely it would be to elicit stuttering.

Taylor (1966b) also reported that the position of a word in a sentence was significantly related to the amount of stuttering that occurred.

This evidence strongly suggests the probability that stuttering is related to the position of the word in the sentence, even when the factors of length of word, initial sound and grammatical form are controlled.

(d) Length of word

Brown and Moren (1942) reported a significant relationship between word length and frequency of stuttering. The same effect was found by Taylor (1966b) to be independent of both position and initial sound effect, but to be less pronounced than either.

It does appear that longer words are more likely to elicit stuttering than shorter words. Some of the discrepant results of the other experiments mentioned are most probably due to the lack of effective control over the other relevant variables. When such controls are operative, as in Taylor's study, the independent effects as related to frequency of stuttering seem to be, in order of importance, consonant/vowel differences, the position a word occupies in a sentence, the length of the word and grammatical form.

5. *Meaningfulness*

Brown proposed that words beginning a sentence were more difficult for the stutterer because they carried more meaning than those which appeared at the end of the sentence. Conway and Quarrington (1963) argued that if this were the case there would be no decrease in stuttering from first to last word in a series of words where there was little or no meaningful relationship between the individual words. To test this idea they constructed groups of words that varied in their approximation to English, ranging from no meaningful connection between successive words, for example "heroes station majority park manner glass consume" (zero order) to "heroes gain considerable praise in our culture" (text order). Figure 13 shows the mean frequency of stuttering for the critical words in the three types of context in relation to position. As can be seen, both the position and the context in which the words were placed affect the amount of stuttering elicited. So this finding offers some support for Brown's hypothesis and also to some extent for that of Eisenson and Horowitz (1945) when they investigated propositionality or meaningfulness in relation to stuttering.

However, although the amount of stuttering can be seen (in Fig. 13) to decline with lower levels of contextual organization, the position effect is still demonstrable, and there is still a decreasing gradient of stuttering from the first to the last word in a sentence. Quarrington (1965) thought the failure to demonstrate that this decrease was solely related to the information value of the words in the sentence might be due to the rather limited nature of the speech sample studied. He therefore constructed a 95-word piece of prose to test once again the idea that stuttering is related to the amount of meaning conveyed by a word in the sentence. To get the information value of each of the 95 words he used a procedure similar to that developed by Selfridge (Miller, 1951). This requires subjects to guess the first word, after which the word is shown to them and they are required to guess the next word, and so on until the whole passage is visible to them.

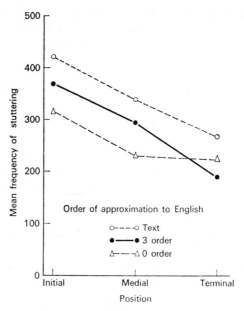

FIG. 13. Mean frequency of stuttering on critical words as a function of position (redrawn from Conway and Quarrington, 1963).

The passage prepared in this way was then read aloud by 24 adult stutterers. The correlation between frequency of stuttering and predictability of the words was -0.32 ($p < 0.01$), which meant that the more readily predictable was the word, the less likelihood there was that the word would be stuttered. The correlation between word position and word predictability was lower than might have been expected, being only 0.22.

By analysing the data further, Quarrington found that the position of the word in the sentence was a more decisive factor in determining stuttering than word predictability, although the latter plays a part. The partial correlation between word position and stuttering, holding word predictability constant, was -0.45 ($p < 0.001$) and that between predictability and stuttering with word position held constant was $-0\cdot25$ ($p<0\cdot05$).

It seems that, while Brown's "meaningfulness" explanation of the stuttering gradient observed in the reading of sentences is supported, there is some other factor which must be sought to fully account for the position effect.

Schlesinger *et al.* (1965) have also drawn a comparison between Brown's "word weighting" factors and the information load of words in a sentence. To support this comparison they state that (a) the first words in a sentence are, on the whole, less predictable than later words (Aborn *et al.*, 1959), (b) longer words tend to be less frequent in the language than shorter words, (Zipf, 1949), and (c) so-called "content" words (nouns, verbs, adverbs and adjectives) are less predictable than "function" words (Aborn *et al.*, 1959; Nicol and Miller 1959).

They go on to show that stuttering occurs more often on words of low transition probability than on those of high transition probability and this difference is greatest when the words of high information value (low transition probability) were also words that occur more rarely in the language. This is an interesting partial replication of Quarrington's results since the language used here was Hebrew.

On the basis of these results their suggestion that the adaptation effect can be accounted for in terms of transition probabilities seems a reasonable one. Having read the prose passage once, the stutterer is clearly in a better position to predict each word as it occurs. It can therefore be hypothesized that during the adaptation trials the words on which stuttering no longer occurs would be directly related to their information value and familiarity.

Taylor and Taylor (1966) have offered an explanation of the tendency for there to be a decreasing probability of stuttering from first to last words in a sentence, which Quarrington (1965) had shown to be an important factor independent of the actual predictability or information value of the word. Goldman-Eisler (1958) has also shown that normal speakers are more likely to hesitate at places where the uncertainty value of the following word is high. Taylor and Taylor hypothesized that these places are ordinarily difficult for the normal speaker and, if a person is prone to stuttering, these are the places where it will occur. However, stuttering is determined not only by the information value of the following word but also by the fact that certain types of position in a sentence tend to have particular degrees of uncertainty (Aborn *et al.*, 1959).

If this is so then it offers further support for the notion that the stutterer is not qualitatively different from the nonstutterer, but only quantitatively. That is, he is more likely to experience disfluencies when confronted with a word in a certain position in a sentence which has high information value, than if that word is in another part of the sentence, and so on.

6. *Conclusions*

1. Words that are stuttered in previous passages will be stuttered on subsequent readings of that passage with more than chance expectancy.

2. The degree of consistency of stuttering is highly related to severity of stuttering.

3. The percentage measure is unsatisfactory. The most flexible and easiest to compute is the "normal deviate score" and tests of significance can be used with this score.

4. Stutterers are able to predict with great accuracy the words on which they will stutter.

5. The occurrence of stuttering appears to be dependent upon the information value of the word and the degree of uncertainty of the position in the sentence that it occupies.

6. The stutterer may be more likely to stutter in those places where the normal speaker is likely to hesitate or pause.

B. THE ADAPTATION EFFECT

1. *Description*

The first description of the adaptation phenomenon has usually been attributed to Johnson and Knott (1937) but it seems to have been observed prior to this (Van Riper and Hull, 1934) in a paper which was not published until 1955.

Among the various definitions of the adaptation effect that have been offered there are the following: to Jones (1955) it is "a decrement in stuttering frequency" (i.e. experimental extinction) (p. 226); to Johnson (1955) it is "the decrease in stuttering as measured with reference to its frequency or severity, that occurs when a stutterer reads the same passage a number of times successively" (p. 15); to

Gray (1965a) it is "a continuing adjustment process of the organism to an ongoing constant stimulus situation" (p. 180).

Whichever proves to be the most satisfactory level of definition, the phenomenon can generally be said to involve the notions of time, and of speaking or reading aloud. At a descriptive level it means that stuttering in the individual tends to reduce in frequency with speaking or reading on several occasions under relatively constant environmental conditions.

This effect has largely been studied *in vacuo* with little attempt to relate it to other phenomena, type of treatment or prognosis. Two exceptions to this statement are the suggested therapeutic implications of the phenomenon offered by Brutten and Gray (1961) and Shames (1953).

The main practical result of research in this area has been to force investigators to "control for the adaptation effect" in any experiment involving the elicitation of repeated responses from the stuttering subject.

The independent variables that have been experimentally investigated in adaptation experiments can broadly be divided into (i) the type and quantity of reading material, (ii) the time interval between oral performances and (iii) environmental conditions under which the oral performance takes place.

2. *Methods of Eliciting Oral Performance*

Before discussing investigations of these independent variables a few words must be said about the manner in which speech is elicited. The vast majority of experiments have used oral reading as the situation for eliciting speech and thereby stuttering, and only a few have tried to measure the effect during spontaneous speech. This is hardly surprising when one realizes how much easier it is to bring the phenomenon under experimental control if previously selected prose passages are used.

Earlier research had in fact suggested that the adaptation obtained in successive oral readings not only failed to transfer to the subsequent spontaneous speech of stutterers (Harris, 1940) but that adaptation in spontaneous speech did not occur at all (Cohen, 1952). Further research has, however, tended to contradict these findings. For example, when Newman (1954) compared oral reading adaptation with that observed in spontaneous speech elicited during the descriptions of drawings, he found that reduction in severity level is common to both oral reading and spontaneous speech, as can be seen in Fig. 14.

The measurement of stuttering severity is fraught with difficulties which have already been discussed in Chapter 2, and these difficulties are maximized when rating severity in spontaneous speech. Newman tackled this task by using the Iowa Scale of Severity of Stuttering

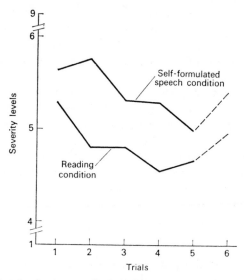

FIG. 14. Trends of mean severity level for six trials under two conditions. The solid lines connect the means for the five successive adaptation trials. The broken lines, connecting the last adaptation trial mean with the recovery trial mean, indicates a 24-hour time interval (redrawn from Newman, 1954).

(Sherman, 1952). He took a recording of each of the consecutive descriptions of drawings, played these back, and made a rating of severity every 10 seconds. The final rating for each speech sample was the mean of these 10-second speech segments. Newman checked for reliability of measurement by correlating his judgements with the scale values established by Sherman (1955), and obtained a correlation of 0·98.

Another check used by Newman was for "word avoidance". He argued that in self-formulated speech there is a tendency for stutterers to avoid words over which they have previously experienced difficulty.

It was therefore possible that an *apparent* increase in adaptation might result. Newman tested this by taking a measure of the consistency with which individual words were stuttered in the first and fifth drawing descriptions and obtained a correlation between this measure of consistency and one of adaptation of $0 \cdot 04$. On the basis of this result he concluded that the adaptation found in self-formulated speech was not a function of "word avoidance".

A marathon study of adaptation in spontaneous speech has also been reported by Rousey (1958) in which subjects' speech was tape-recorded for 10 hours a day for 5 consecutive days. His subjects were 5 girls and 13 boys aged from $13 \cdot 8$ years to $17 \cdot 6$ years. Ratings of severity, presence of secondary symptoms, and number of words spoken, were used as measures and were taken at hourly intervals throughout the day. Significant changes on all three measures occurred during any one day, which is in line with what would be expected if the adaptation effect were operative. Similar results pertained to comparisons between consecutive days, except that the severity measure failed to show a reduction in stuttering during the course of the 5 days. The author observes that in fact two subjects stuttered more at the end of their 50 hours of talking than they had at the beginning. It is to be regretted that in this, as in so many other studies, information is given about mean scores but none as to the variance, so that little idea about degree of individual differences can be gained.

3. *Independent Variables Studied*

(a) *The reading material*

Most definitions mention a constancy or stability within the adaptation situation, so that changing the reading material between adaptation trials might be expected to alter the rate and extent of the reduction in stuttering frequency achieved. Thus, in the typical situation, the stutterer is placed in a room with the experimenter and is instructed to read aloud a passage of some 100–200 words and, after a pause of a second or two, is asked to repeat the reading up to a total of five times. The reading passage(s) will usually be constructed in some systematic way, such as containing every speech sound in the initial position of at least one word (Van Riper and Hull, 1955), or else the order of the passages is systematically varied, but such care is by no means invariably found.

The score most commonly used is expressed in the formula $(x-y)/x$, in which x is the frequency or percentage of words stuttered on the first reading and y is the frequency or percentage of words stuttered on the second reading.

It has consistently been reported that in the typical situation just described, there is a reduction in the number of stutters over five successive readings of the same passage of about 50% (e.g. Johnson and Inness, 1939; Trotter, 1955; Jones, 1955), which produces the

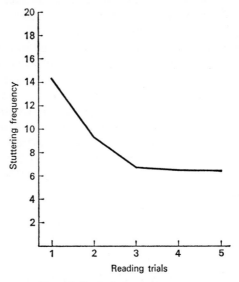

FIG. 15. Typical adaptation curve.

typical curve shown in Fig. 15. However, when the material differs from trial to trial, less than 20% reduction in stuttering is found (e.g. Johnson and Inness, 1939; Golud, 1955). The Johnson and Inness material consisted of a whole passage of prose divided up into segments with no pause between each segment, and Donohue (1955) adopted this method when he studied the adaptation effect in subjects reading aloud for 3 hours without a pause. He found that the mean errors per minute dropped from 3·0 during the first hour, to 1·6 during the third. This reduction in disfluencies cannot be attributed solely to fatigue since it is similar in amount to that found in other experiments. However, fatigue may well play some part since Curtis (1942) reported a reduction in stuttering to occur with fatigue produced by muscular exercise, and he suggests that an increase in stuttering under these conditions might be expected by those supporting some type of neurophysiological theory of the aetiology of stuttering.

At first sight it would seem that this reduction in frequency of stuttering with changing reading material has not always been demonstrated. For instance, Wischner (1952) obtained results that, at face value, were the opposite to Donohue's (Fig. 16), but he goes

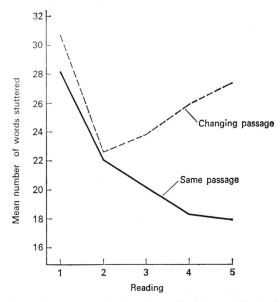

FIG. 16. The effect on stuttering behaviour of varying specific word anxiety in successive readings. The solid line represents the usual stuttering adaptation curve obtained with successive readings of the same material. The dotted line shows the relative effect of changing passages at each reading (redrawn from Wischner, 1952).

on to show that this is not so. He calculated the frequency of stuttering of Donohue's subjects over the first five 200-word segments and found that the "mean number of words stuttered by 10 Ss in each 200-word segment was as follows: $17 \cdot 8$, $11 \cdot 8$, $9 \cdot 1$, $14 \cdot 7$ and $14 \cdot 5$". A plot of these means yielded a curve of the same general shape, with initial sharp drop and subsequent increase. Wischner suggests that the reason why the subsequent increase in stuttering is not regular in Donohue's study is that the reading material was continuous, and so the subject was not presented with a new passage to begin each time. By beginning a new passage each time Wischner feels the subject is responding to specific word anxiety after the initial reduction in situational anxiety. This does not seem to explain very satisfactorily why the increase in stuttering after the second trial is so steady, and seemingly would continue to be so.

In addition to these studies designed to show the relative effects of using the same or different passages at each reading, Shulman (1955) looked to see if the *length* of reading material had any effect on the amount of resulting adaptation. She found that it made no appreciable difference to the adaptation curve whether the passage was of 200, 500 or 1000 words. It also seems to make little difference whether lists of words are used instead of the usual prose passage (Golud, 1955).

One last experiment of importance, to do with the material which the subject is required to read within the adaptation situation, is that of Van Riper and Hull (1955). These authors attempted to isolate whether the adaptation was a function of familiarity with the syntax and structure of the reading material or with the situation. They first obtained adaptation scores for subjects over a number of readings and then had them read the 133-word passage *backwards*. They found no great increase in number of speech errors, nor was there much increase when the words of the passage were rearranged. They thus concluded that the adaptation must be to the situation rather than to the passage. To test this the subjects were required to read a passage until a stable plateau of "stutters" had been reached, then to read into a microphone, and then to an audience of strangers. Ninety-five per cent of the subjects exhibited an increase in number of "stutters" in both situations.

(b) *Time intervals between readings*

Shulman (1955) used zero, 15 minutes, 30 minutes and 24 hours as intervals between successive readings of the same passage and found the amount of adaptation to be inversely related to the length of the interval, that is, the greatest reduction in stuttering occurred when no interval between readings was used. It is also interesting to note in this experiment that, with a 24-hour interval, *more* stuttering on average occurred when the first reading was compared with the second, third and fourth readings and that the intersubject variability was very large indeed. In spite of this, a significant reduction in frequency of stuttering was demonstrated between the first and fifth 24-hour trial.

The same general finding was reported by Leutenegger (1957) in an experiment using time intervals of 20, 60 minutes and 24 hours between each of five trials, each trial consisting of two readings. The mean frequency of the stutters on each of these readings can be seen in Fig. 17. Leutenegger found that a reduction in stuttering occurred

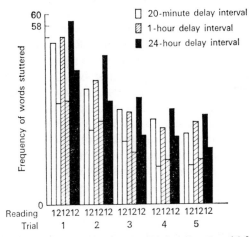

FIG. 17. Mean frequency of words stuttered in readings 1 and 2 for each of the 5 trials in each of the recovery delay interval conditions (redrawn from Leutenegger, 1957).

over each time interval and also that the amount of adaptation tended to decrease with increasing intervals. These two experiments differed in that Shulman measured adaptation on the basis of one reading per trial and Leutenegger measured on the basis of two readings so the results cannot be directly compared.

(c) The environmental situation

The previously discussed study of Van Riper and Hull stimulated an interest in the effects of environmental factors on the amount of adaptation occurring. It must be remembered that the study was carried out in 1934 although not published until 1955.

One of the areas of interest has been the effect on adaptation of the number of people present during the sessions. Porter (1939), for instance, increased the size of the audience at each successive reading and found that the frequency of stuttering varied directly with the increase in audience size. Contradictory results were then reported by Shulman (1955), who found that adaptation still occurred when the size of the audience was steadily increased. Shulman attributes these differences to the facts that the change in audience size in his experiment was brought about more gradually than Porter's and that he used the *same* reading material in each trial while Porter used *different* passages.

The difference in percentage adaptation between having only the experimenter present and having an audience is similar to that reported when the same and different passages are used for oral reading, i.e. 46·0% and 20·44% respectively between first and fifth readings. When a condition involving speaking into a field telephone was used (Dixon, 1955) still less adaptation resulted. One way of reconciling the differences obtained by Porter and Shulman is suggested by Wischner's idea (1952) that there is anxiety attached to both words *and* situations. Thus Porter was using conditions which might be expected to keep word and situation anxiety at a maximum, whereas Shulman was allowing a decrease in *word* anxiety and so producing a situation in which adaptation might be expected to occur.

Siegel and Haugen (1964) argue that the greatest amount of adaptation should result when reading material is held constant and the size of the audience is systematically decreased. To test this they used three audience conditions—a constant audience, an audience which progressively increased in size (a replication of Shulman's study), and a progressively decreasing audience. Unfortunately, the subjects in the "increasing" and "decreasing" groups differed significantly in initial frequency of stuttering. This meant that any cross-group comparisons were invalid because of the ample evidence that amount of adaptation is negatively correlated with initial frequency of stuttering. They were able, however, to compare each condition with its own control (a constant audience of one) and found that adaptation did occur with increase in audience size but less so than in the control group. Likewise, the decreasing audience produced adaptation, but only the same amount as that found in the control situation (see Fig. 18).

An experiment by Young (1965) has a direct bearing on this

hypothesized correlation between audience size and frequency of stuttering, although it is not an investigation of adaptation itself. Young's subjects read different passages on consecutive days to audiences of from one to four people. He argued that stutterers can predict the degree to which they will stutter in a given situation. In most previous experiments relating audience size to frequency of stuttering, audience size has been systematically increased or decreased so that the subject has been able to "evaluate the expected

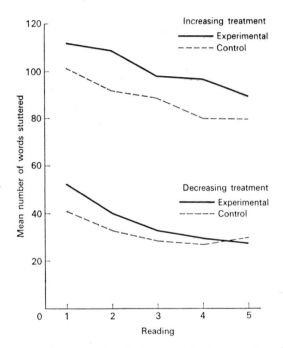

FIG. 18. Mean frequency of stuttering on each of five readings for Increasing and Decreasing audience size treatment groups, in the control and experimental conditions for each treatment (redrawn from Siegel and Haugen, 1964).

difficulty, and behave accordingly" (p. 401). To overcome this Young randomly varied the order of speakers, reading passage and audience size. Each speaker read only once on each of 4 days and there was no increase in stuttering with an increase in audience size.

If audience size is not related to frequency of stuttering, then the differences in results obtained by various experimenters in amount of adaptation recorded must be a function of other variables, such as reading material and time intervals.

4. *Scoring*

Quarrington (1959) has expressed dissatisfaction with the percentage adaptation measurement that has been traditionally used. He points out that a measure that correlates $-0 \cdot 40$ to $-0 \cdot 65$ with initial frequency is unsatisfactory since the considerable intra-individual variation in stuttering severity will result in a lowering of reliability. Also, Tate *et al.* (1961) state that it is statistically unclear how to average percentage adaptation scores, that distributions of such scores are irregularly rectangular, and that in 5 out of 6 of the samples studied the distributions were bimodal with the modes at or near the extremes.

To overcome these difficulties Quarrington (1959) suggested a residual measure of adaptation based on a deviation from a regression line that would be independent of initial frequency. Tate and his associates compared this score, the percentage score and two other measures, and found that the percentage score was the least satisfactory and that the other three measures correlated very highly with each other. Which of these three latter scores should be used depends, in their opinion, on the use to which the score is to be put.

5. *Reliability*

Recent studies have demonstrated that the stability of the adaptation phenomenon is to some extent a function of the measure used. For instance, Liebman (1956) reports a test–retest correlation for the percentage score of $0 \cdot 68$ over a 2-week period, Quarrington (1959) obtained a correlation of $0 \cdot 69$ for the residual score and $0 \cdot 42$ for the percentage score, while Cullinan (1963) reports correlations of $0 \cdot 64$ for the residual score and $0 \cdot 35$ for the percentage score. Cullinan investigated reliability further by removing all data for subjects exhibiting less than 2% stuttered words on the first reading of the first day. As a result of this the percentage score test–retest correlation rose to $0 \cdot 70$, while those for other scores remained substantially unchanged.

In addition to the rather low test–retest correlations, Cullinan found very large standard errors of measurement. From this he concluded that a single adaptation score or a mean of three such scores cannot be taken as representative of the stutterer's speech behaviour. This finding must inevitably present a difficulty to those who would wish to use such scores for prognostic purposes, or as measures of therapeutic improvement.

Cullinan then went on to see whether measures of adaptation using overall reading rate and nonstuttered reading rate would be more stable. However, he again found large standard errors of measurement over three adaptation trials and concluded that these are also too unstable to be used as a measure of an individual's performance.

6. *Expectancy and Adaptation*

Another section of this review has dealt with experiments designed to show that subjects are able to anticipate which words they will have difficulty in speaking (Chapter 3). Wischner (1952) wondered whether the adaptation phenomenon might be demonstrable with expectancy of stuttering and whether, if it were, it would vary as a function of the time interval between successive inspections of the same material. To test this he first of all had subjects inspect a passage of prose once each day for 5 days and underline words on which they would expect to stutter. Four days later they had to mark a second passage on five separate occasions, but this time with no time interval between the five inspections. Figure 19 shows that with no interval between readings a typical reduction in anticipated stutterings occurred, whereas with 24-hour intervals the curve was totally different.

Peins (1961), however, failed to find any evidence of an expectancy adaptation effect resulting from five successive silent readings of the same passage with zero interval between readings which were repeated on 4 successive days. She suggests three possible factors which might have lead to this failure to replicate Wischner's finding; (a) her subjects were older, having a mean age of 22·2 years to Wischner's 18 years (Harris (1942) found that stutterers below 18 years of age adapted more rapidly and to a greater extent than did the adults), (b) her subjects were tested individually and Wischner's in a group, and (c) her stutterers had not acted as subjects in research projects before, whereas Wischner's had taken part in several previous adaptation experiments, which could well have led them to "be prepared" to adapt.

Brutten (1963) had stutterers and nonstutterers underline words on which they might expect difficulty if they were to read them aloud. As well as this he took a palmar sweat print as a measure of anxiety adaptation for both groups at the first, third and fifth readings. He found oral adaptation to occur in both stutterers and nonstutterers, but for only the stutterers did the palmar sweat scores covary with the adaptation scores, trial by trial. Regarding expectancy adaptation, this was demonstrated for the nonstutterers on both physiological

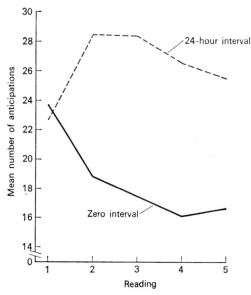

FIG. 19. The mean number of anticipations marked by Ss during five successive inspections of the same material in Condition I (24-hour interval between inspections) and condition 2 (zero interval between inspections) (redrawn from Wischner, 1952).

and silent reading measures, but for the stutterers the median expectancy of stuttering did not differ from first to fifth trial, nor did the median palmar sweat scores. It is difficult on the basis of these results to account for Brutten's summary that "(a) stutterers and nonstutterers show disfluency and expectancy adaptation during massed oral and silent readings, (b) disfluency and expectancy adaptation of the stutterers is associated with a covarying decrease in palmar sweat scores". It is suggested that if one uses statistical techniques to calculate whether or not a given difference in scores occurred by chance, then one should abide by the minimal level of significance generally accepted, unless one shows good reason why a lower level is preferred.

Failure to find the expectancy effect once again could be due to the fact that, like Peins' subjects, Brutten's were naïve and were tested individually rather than in a group. He does not report the age of his subjects so the relevance of this variable cannot be assessed.

7. The Transfer of Adaptation

From the various experiments that have been discussed in this section and in the section dealing with spontaneous recovery, it is possible to glean some information about the extent to which any adaptation that has occurred persists over time and is transferable from one situation to another and from one type of speaking situation to another. For instance, Peins' (1961) data show that there is a progressive decrease in stuttering frequency at the first reading on each of 4 successive days, indicating some carry-over of adaptation when there is a 24-hour interval between any five adaptation readings. Leutenegger (1957) also obtained similar results with 24 hours between sessions as is shown in Fig. 17, the first trial on each day producing less stuttering than the first trial on the previous day.

There were some earlier indications (e.g. Harris, 1942) that adaptation could be transferred from one passage of prose to another over short time intervals, but not from prose to conversational speech. Gray and Brutten (1965) were unable to find any such carry-over of adaptation, and one possible explanation of this discrepancy could be sought in Harris' finding that his younger subjects adapted more easily and this carried over to another passage more readily than for the adults. He says that "the older stutterers in this experiment have apparently fixated their reactions more on individual sounds and 'difficult' words than have the younger group, thus bringing about a slower rate of adaptation" (p. 217).

8. Adaptation in the Listener and the Nonstutterer

While most of the literature has centred around the study of the adaptation phenomenon in stutterers, there have been a few attempts to compare it with that found in the disfluencies of nonstutterers and to discuss the theoretical implications of this.

Starbuck and Steer (1953) found the effect to be present in both stutterers and nonstutterers but reported there to be a significant difference in the shape of the adaptation curve. They concluded that, although the effect was present in both groups, it was not the same.

Investigating this further, Gray (1965a) demonstrated curves for the two groups of subjects to be similar to those found by Starbuck

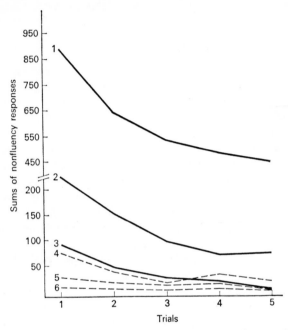

FIG. 20. Nonfluency adaptation continuum for mild, moderate and severe stutterers and nonstutterers. 1 = severe stutterers; 2 = moderate stutterers; 3 = mild stutterers; 4 = severe nonstutterers; 5 = moderate nonstutterers; and 6 = mild nonstutterers (redrawn from Gray, 1965a).

and Steer, but questioned their conclusions that the curves were qualitatively different. He subdivided each group into "severe", "moderate" and "mild" and the resulting adaptation curves for these subgroups can be seen in Fig. 20. Both "severe" stutterers and non-stutterers have relatively steep curves while "moderate" and "mild" stutterers have relatively flat ones.

In another study, Gray and Karmen (1966) isolated differences between stutterers and nonstutterers during adaptation by subdividing them into "high", "moderate" and "low" on the basis of (a) number of disfluencies and (b) palmar sweat index score. They found that the "moderate" stutterer had a significantly higher palmar sweat index than the other two subgroups, but there were no such subgroup differences for the nonstutterer. Also, the "moderate" palmar sweat index stutterer subgroup had significantly lower levels of disfluency adaptation, which again was not found with the nonstutterers. These results lead the authors to suggest that the assumed correlation between severity of stuttering and general anxiety level may need to be re-examined. That intragroup differences were found among stutterers and not among nonstutterers implies that there may be qualitative as well as quantitative differences between the groups as a whole, or that some subgroups of stutterers can be placed along the same continuum as nonstutterers while others cannot. A further explanation might be that the number of disfluencies among the "normal" speakers are too few to allow subgroup differences to emerge.

Gray has suggested that the adaptation phenomenon is a reflection of an adjustment process of the individual to a constant stimulus situation. He also hypothesized (1965a) that the depth of the curve is a function of the initial frequency of stuttering. To investigate this he calculated regression equations for predicting the number of "stutters" on a subsequent trial from the number elicited on the first trial. Using his table of approximations (Gray 1965a, pp. 221–7) the predicted scores for each adaptation trial correlated from 0·92 to 0·99 with the obtained score in all cases except one, where the correlation was 0·84.

It is interesting that the data used for making these predictions were selected from previous studies that had employed very different experimental conditions, for example with and without drugs, with and without an audience. Although the correlations between predicted and obtained scores are high, in nearly all cases the mean differences between the actual and predicted portions of the curve are statistically significant and the range of differences is large. So that, although the latter is probably due to one or two extreme scores in the data, as Gray suggests, the prediction for an individual is likely to be somewhat unreliable. However, Gray's aim was not to provide the reader with a statistical equation for predicting an adaptation curve, but to demonstrate the lawfulness of the phenomenon. Gray's results suggest that previous studies that have sought to manipulate supposed independent variables may simply have been manipulating the initial frequency of stuttering.

Gray also applied his table of approximations to the prediction of scores for the group of 33 nonstutterers over five trials (personal communication), with the results given in Table 10.

TABLE 10

To show obtained and predicted number of nonfluencies for a group of 33 nonstutterers using the Table of Approximations (Gray, 1965b)

	Adaptation trials				
	1	2	3	4	5
Sum of obtained nonfluencies	125	87	51	48	38
Sum of predicted nonfluencies	—	99	88	79	90

One reason suggested by Gray for the poor fit between actual and predicted scores is that 23 of the sample had disfluencies of under 5 on the first reading trial and, since the table of approximations starts with an initial score of 5, two-thirds of the population were outside the range of the table. The predictive data for this group of nonstutterers with scores above 5, the mean differences and standard errors of the correlations are shown in Table 11.

TABLE 11

To show correlations, mean differences and standard errors of the mean differences between predicted and obtained scores on five adaptation trials for a sample of nonstutterers with more than 5 speech errors using the Table of Approximations (Gray, 1965b)

	Adaptation trials				
	1	2	3	4	5
r	—	0·6	0·45	0·45	—
MD	—	1·2	1·2	1·6	2·4
SE_{MD}	—	1·6	1·1	1·9	—

The rather lower correlations between predicted and actual disfluencies for these nonstutterers is no doubt due to the very restricted range of scores (5–10). Whether or not nonstutterers adapt in the same way as stutterers is thus still in doubt, but Gray suggests that "one way to get at this problem, would be to have a reading task of sufficient size to permit a high enough frequency of fluency failure" (personal communication).

Lastly, he demonstrates very clearly (see Fig. 21) one reason why curves that are proportional to each other have such a different shape. The top curve is utilizing far more of the range of the ordinate than the bottom of the curve although both are plots of the same data.

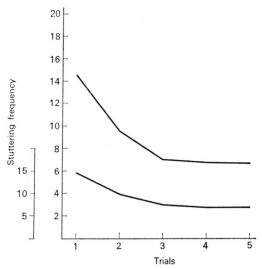

FIG. 21. The same hypothetical adaptation curve plotted on two different ordinates to show change in configuration as a function of scaling methods (redrawn from Gray, 1965a).

From a theoretical point of view Gray's demonstration of the lawfulness of the adaptation phenomenon, irrespective of experimental conditions, is of great interest. He points out that many of the previous studies in which an independent variable has been supposed to produce a qualitative difference in the curve will need to be reassessed to see whether they do in fact contradict this concept of proportionality.

He speculates that adaptation is a reflection of the subject's continuous appraisal of the stimulus situation along a "threat–no threat" dimension, with the initial level of stuttering being determined by how threatening the subject considers the situation to be. However, he is not able to suggest what it is that makes a situation threatening or not threatening to the stutterer.

One finding of Gray's that should not be overlooked is that for 85% of the stutterers the adaptation curve could be predicted with reasonable accuracy, but this was not so for 10% of the sample who yielded a flat or w-shaped curve, and with 5% who had a negative adaptation curve. The significance of these latter unusual curves is not clear but if they are shown to be part of a consistent pattern for the individual then this would add to St. Onge's contention (1964) that stuttering is not a single disorder. This idea is given further support by Gray and Karmen's (1966) findings. They subdivided a group of stutterers in terms of number of disfluencies and found the "moderate" subgroup to have significantly higher anxiety scores on all five adaptation trials, and the anxiety adaptation curve for the "moderate" subgroup also differed significantly from the other two.

In an attempt to highlight the individual differences in relation to the adaptation effect, Newman (1963) reanalysed some previous group data. When the adaptation was measured for reading and self-formulated speech, 6 out of 20 stutterers did not adapt in the former situation, while 7 out of 20 failed to adapt in the latter. For these cases all but one *increased* in stuttering severity from trials 1 to 5. Only one of the subjects failed to adapt in both situations. Newman suggests that stutterers could be subdivided according to their ability to adapt and then tested on other behavioural measures. It would be interesting to compare the adaptation curves of, for instance, each of Goldiamond's (1965) stutterers with those found by Gray and by Newman.

9. *Adaptation, Prognosis and Therapy*

One of the few practical attempts to use the knowledge about this phenomenon has been to try to relate it to success in therapy. Johnson (1956) saw the supposed lawfulness of the effect as a "laboratory model of the improvement process" (p. 257) and the idea has been tested experimentally by Lanyon (1965). He hypothesized that high adaptation and low consistency would be positively correlated with improvement in stuttering therapy. Because of Cullinan's finding that different methods of scoring had different reliabilities, Lanyon used both the percentage and residual scores. He also took the precaution of partialling out initial severity when calculating the percentage score because of the high negative correlation between the two. He found that two of the three improvement scores (clinician ratings and increase in speaking rate) were significantly correlated with percentage scores but none were related to residual adaptation scores or consistency scores. The significant correlations increased (to 0·60 and 0·40 respectively) when corrected for unreliability, but Lanyon concluded that these are not sufficiently high for clinical use.

On present evidence it thus seems that a relationship between clinical improvement and adaptation scores exists but that it is not sufficiently close to be of use as a clinical predictor. Gray (personal communication) is at present conducting some research in which he is attempting to isolate different types of stutterers and then relating the scores obtained by these subgroups on various measures (including adaptation) to type of therapy and prognosis.

Although he did not provide any experimental evidence to support his suggestion, Shames (1953) described a way in which the adaptation effect could be utilized in the treatment of stuttering. The stutterer is first adapted to a passage of prose and then deliberately produces stuttering speech (negative practice). By doing this the problem of the appearance of "real" stuttering blocks is minimized. Having adapted to the situation and the prose, and successfully carried out the negative practice, this whole procedure is repeated in gradually changing situations. This general type of procedure would now be subsumed under the heading of "behaviour therapy" or "deconditioning", but Shames' account is of interest in its deliberate and systematic use of the adaptation effect.

10. *Theories of Adaptation*

Wischner (1950) hypothesized that stuttering is learned behaviour reinforced by anxiety reduction, so that when the reinforcing agent is no longer present extinction of the learned response occurs. Adaptation is thus analogous to experimental extinction. Interesting though this might be at first sight, it is an explanation the validity of which cannot at present be tested. To do so it would be necessary to identify the nature of the reinforcing agent that normally keeps the stuttering behaviour going and the omission of which would lead to the extinction of the response. Jones (1955), Leutenegger (1957) as well as Wischner himself have all underlined this difficulty and it therefore seems rather unprofitable to continue using this as a theoretical explanation of the adaptation effect until such time as the reinforcer can be described.

Johnson and his colleagues (1956) see adaptation as resulting from a reduction in anxiety which occurs when things have not turned out as badly as the stutterer thought they were going to be.

> With less intense anxiety, he is subsequently less apprehensive about stuttering on the words he has to say, less concerned about avoiding the stuttering he does anticipate, and so he does less to avoid it and does it with less tension. For this essential reason there is adaptation; that is, more and more talking leads to less and less stuttering because the stutterer gradually learns that, in general, his expectations are exaggerated and that speaking is nearly always not as bad as he thinks it will be.

In an experiment already discussed, Peins (1961) argues that Wischner's experimental extinction analogy and Johnson's theory of anxiety deconfirmation both depend on the occurrence of overt stuttering, so that if the adaptation effect could be demonstrated during silent reading, which then carried over to reading aloud, this would provide invalidating evidence for both explanations. However, she failed to find any reduction in stuttering expectancy during the silent reading trials 1 to 5 on any of 4 consecutive days, yet on the reading aloud trials on the fourth day a fairly typical adaptation curve was obtained. Because of the failure of the expectancy phenomenon to occur the experiment could not be considered to be a real test of any carry-over of adaptation from the silent to the aloud situation.

Unlike the experimental extinction explanation, the anxiety reduction hypothesis as formulated by Johnson more readily lends itself to experimental test. In an experiment previously mentioned, Brutten (1963) found significant reductions in frequency of stuttering and palmar sweat scores purporting to measure anxiety during oral reading. In a later study Gray and Brutten (1965) failed to find a similar covariance over adaptation trials, that is, the palmar sweat scores did not increase and decrease to mirror similar changes in stuttering frequency. In a personal communication Gray offers a possible reason for the discrepant results. In Brutten's study the subject was presented with a packet of reading passages stapled together. The subject was instructed to read each page and then turn to the next, which was identical. He continued in this way throughout the session. In the Gray and Brutten study, the subject was given one page and told to read it. The page was taken away after it had been read and another identical page handed to him. Gray suggests that in the former study the subject could form a "gestalt" whereas in the latter he was uncertain of the limits of the experiment. He concludes that the anxiety reduction found by Brutten may have been an arte-fact of the experimental procedure.

Hull's (1943) construct of reactive inhibition has been invoked by several writers to explain the reduction in stuttering with repetition (e.g. Wischner, 1947; Luper, 1954; Brutten, 1957; Gray and Brutten, 1965). Reactive inhibition in the Hullian system is a negative drive.

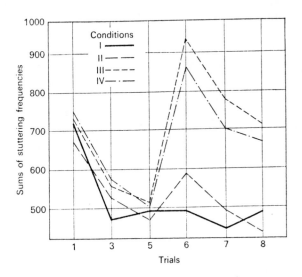

FIG. 22. Stuttering frequencies over 8 trials under 4 conditions (Gray and Brutten, 1965).

If a response is constantly repeated, with little time allowed between trials for recovery, there is a build-up of reactive inhibition and the activity is weakened.

Gray and Brutten suggest that there is a build-up of both reactive inhibition (I_R) and conditioned inhibition ($_sI_R$) during the reading of the same passage over five massed trials. That is to say, during continuous elicitation of stuttering I_R accumulates and becomes a drive toward rest. When a rest or cessation of stuttering occurs, the drive is reduced by the dissipation of the I_R. However, like other conditioned responses, and unlike reactive inhibition, $_sI_R$ would not dissipate during rest; according to theory it would be expected to persist and to produce a permanent work decrement.

Figure 22 shows that on the sixth trial (trials 1–5 being reading the same passage with 20-second intervals) there was (a) no change when reading was done under the same conditions as for trials 1–5 (condition I); (b) there was an increase in stuttering frequency following a 7-minute interval (condition II); and (c) there was a similar increase in stuttering to above initial frequency level when a new passage was read but no rest pause given (condition III); and (d) when both a new passage was read and a 7-minute rest pause given (condition IV). These findings tend to suggest that I_R and $_sI_R$ are related specifically to the reading material. This is contrary to Van Riper and Hull's results in which no increase in stuttering was reported when the adaptation passage was read backwards or when the words were rearranged. It could be argued that Van Riper and Hill used the same words in their different conditions and that I_R is built up to these specific words regardless of order or meaningfulness, in which case no increase in stuttering frequency would be predicted. Whereas, although no doubt there were some words common to both the Gray and Brutten passages, the majority would be different.

The importance placed upon the need for establishing the degree of stimulus specificity of I_R build-up depends on the extent to which the concept is of theoretical and therapeutic value. If reactive inhibition and the consequent conditioned inhibition were shown to be markedly dependent on specific words and environmental stimuli, this would explain the difficulty in obtaining generalization of improvement from the therapeutic situation to the "everyday world outside". This question of inhibition will be discussed again in the section on spontaneous recovery.

Peins (1961) briefly suggests an alternative hypothesis to account for the adaptation effect, although she does not regard it as incompatible with previous explanations. Her suggestion is that "material read aloud by the stutterer becomes nonpropositional or meaningless in nature with successive readings". While there is evidence to show that frequency of stuttering is related to communicative responsibility, as has been discussed at the beginning of this chapter, it would be difficult to invoke this notion to explain the some 20% reduction consistently reported when different material is read on each trial. Also, can it be assumed that with continuous reading, or with conversational speech, that the reduction in stuttering, sometimes reported, results from what the person says or reads becoming more meaningless or less important?

11. *Conclusions*

1. The adaptation effect, or reduction in stuttering, has been reliably demonstrated to occur when the same passage of prose or list of words is read a number of times, when no interval or an interval of a few minutes separates each reading.

2. Adaptation has sometimes been demonstrated to occur during spontaneous speech or continuous reading.

3. Changes in the experimental adaptation situation may serve only to alter the initial level of stuttering.

4. It is possible to predict the slope of the adaptation curve for a group, given the frequency of stuttering on the first trial. Prediction for the individual is unlikely to be very reliable due to the relatively large standard errors.

5. Initial frequency of stuttering is negatively correlated with amount of adaptation.

6. The commonly used percentage scoring measure is far less satisfactory than the residual normal deviate or trend measure (for details of these scores see Tate *et al.*, 1961).

7. Whatever score is used, test–retest reliabilities are too low for a single adaptation trial to be taken as a measure of an individual's performance.

8. No definite conclusions can be drawn as to whether the adaptation found with nonstutterers' disfluencies is qualitatively different from that found with stutterers. However, the adaptation effect has been demonstrated in both groups, although subgroup differences have been noted in relation to anxiety level.

9. None of the existing theories of the adaptation effect have been sufficiently investigated for final conclusions to be drawn.

10. The adaptation effect is still largely of academic interest only, although sporadic attempts have been made to integrate it into treatment programmes and to use it to assess prognosis.

11. By no means all stutterers yield a typical adaptation curve. It has been suggested that groups be subdivided in terms of their ability to adapt, and then tested to see whether they can be similarly differentiated on other variables.

C. SPONTANEOUS RECOVERY

1. *Description*

Just as there is a lawful decrease in stuttering with repeated reading aloud, so there is a tendency for the frequency of stuttering to increase to its former level after a delay period. This is hardly surprising since, if there were no "relapse", the use of adaptation as a basis of treatment would be universal.

This increase in frequency of stuttering subsequent to an experimentally induced decrease has been termed "spontaneous recovery" and was first systematically described by Wischner in 1947. As its name suggests, it has often been viewed as a phenomenon similar to that found in Pavlovian conditioning. That is, when a conditioned response has been subjected to extinction trials it will spontaneously return to its full strength following a time interval.

2. *Experimental Evidence*

Jamison (1955) demonstrated that the stuttering response increased following adaptation as a function of the rest interval. There had been 55% recovery of the response after $\frac{1}{2}$ hour, 63·4% after $1\frac{1}{2}$ hours and was fully reinstated after a $4\frac{1}{2}$-hour interval.

The relationship between amount of recovery and interval after adaptation trials was investigated further by Leutenegger (1957). He used trials consisting of two readings of the same material to produce the adaptation effect, the trials being separated by different time intervals; 20 minutes (condition 1), 60 minutes (condition 2) and 24 hours (condition 3). Each condition consisted of 5 trials. Histograms of the frequency of stuttering can be seen in Fig. 17. The amount of recovery was proportionately the same under each delay interval but within each condition there were increasing amounts of adaptation and spontaneous recovery from trial 1 to trial 5.

Frick (1955) set out to investigate this relationship between spontaneous recovery and number of prior adaptation trials. Unfortunately, one cannot unequivocally accept his conclusions that degree of recovery is unaffected by the number of adaptation trials, because the data on which he performed the analysis of variance are highly skewed. The use of parametric statistics on data whose distributions are not normal is a frequent occurrence in the reporting of experiments on stuttering, particularly the early ones, and this must always be borne in mind when assessing the author's conclusions. As an example, Frick's means and standard deviations for his "recovery" trials are given in Table 12.

TABLE 12

To show means and standard deviations for five "recovery" trials (Frick, 1955)

Mean			Standard deviation	
Trial	I	II	I	II
1	33·95	24·25	34·54	29·55
2	27·75	24·05	35·62	28·90
3	25·70	21·70	34·41	27·81
4	25·50	20·75	34·63	29·08
5	25·40	19·85	36·01	27·42

From a theoretical point of view Gray and Brutten (1965) argue that "since adaptation and recovery appear to be functionally related (Gray, 1961; Meikle, 1962) factors which are considered antecedent to adaptation have been considered to be antecedent to spontaneous recovery". In their experiment, reported in some detail in the last section, they found no evidence to support the contention that adaptation and spontaneous recovery are related to changes in anxiety drive level. They thus favour an explanation that spontaneous recovery is a direct consequence of the dissipation of inhibition during the time interval.

Having just noted the use of parametric statistics on skewed data, it is pertinent to mention that Gray and Brutten use non-parametric statistics throughout "since a population of stutterers cannot be considered as being normally distributed."

3. *Conclusions*

1. The reinstatement of the stuttering response has been reliably shown to occur following an interval subsequent to adaptation trials.

2. The frequency of stuttering may return to its initial level some $4\frac{1}{2}$ hours after the adaptation trials.

3. There is no evidence that the amount of recovery is a function of the number of preceding adaptation trials.

4. One theory of spontaneous recovery supported by experimental evidence is that it is a result of the dissipation of reactive inhibition during the interval separating the recovery trials from the adaptation trials.

CHAPTER 7

STUDIES OF DELAYED AUDITORY FEEDBACK, THE "RHYTHM EFFECT", AND OPERANT CONDITIONING, IN THE MODIFICATION OF STUTTERING

1. *Introduction*

In this chapter three important procedures which have been used as techniques for the modification of stuttering are discussed. They are of special interest not simply because they have particular relevance for treatment, but primarily because they represent fairly radically different approaches to the problems of modification and control of nonfluencies. The procedures are not obviously logically related although they may, at some stage of research development, be found to share common ground and, indeed, suggestions have been made that "masking" and the "rhythm effect" are linked by a common mechanism in the context of stuttering control. However, their separate origins and their different development and experimental backgrounds help to preserve a useful "broad front" approach to research in this field.

In the case of "masking" procedures the impetus to current research owes much to the work on delayed auditory feedback of Cherry and Sayers, and implications of perceptual defect in stuttering and the possibility of "organic" aetiology in this disorder are contained in their approach. On the other hand, the "rhythm effect" derives from a lengthy history of empirical observation, and its survival in current therapy and research is attributable to its power to influence stuttering rather than to any carefully worked, coherent theoretical structure concerning its mode of operation. In the case of operant conditioning, we find that its application to stuttering phenomena simply represents a logical extension of basic principles and findings to an area of behaviour not previously covered, and to which these principles and facts appear to be appropriate.

The important consideration which one might have in mind in evaluating work carried out in terms of these three approaches, is that only a beginning has been made, and a great deal is left to be done. It is fortunate that exploration in these avenues of research continues to flourish and expand with an emphasis upon systematic and controlled experimentation.

2. *Experimental Studies of D.A.F. and Masking*

The method of using delayed auditory feedback (D.A.F.) to produce speech disturbances among normally speaking persons was first described by Lee (1950). The method involved recording the speaker's verbal output and playing this back to him with a delay of $\frac{1}{15}$ to $\frac{1}{10}$ second. Very often the result of using this technique is that of considerable disruption of speech behaviour over which the speaker has very little control; blocking, prolongation (i.e. drawing out the length of words), hesitancies, and so on, occur to a marked degree. Using a variety of feedback delay intervals these effects have been noted and confirmed by a number of independent observers.

As Cherry and Sayers point out (1956), Kern (1932) had emphasized the importance of feedback in auditory perception and its possible implications for stuttering, and had described what occurred as a result of having stutterers read aloud to the accompaniment of a loud noise. Kern, however, had attached little therapeutic significance to the observation that "deafening" the stutterer produced striking increases in fluency, while Cherry and Sayers not only conducted a series of excellent experiments into the mechanisms involved in D.A.F., but recognized that the defective feedback hypothesis carried important implications for the treatment of stuttering.

In their paper they point out that imitative speech behaviour may perhaps be related to phenomena such as yawning, giggling and other imitative responses, in the sense that it appears to be "natural" and easily evoked. Shadowing (i.e. monitoring aloud what is being said by some other person) appears to be "imitative" in this special sense, and it has the important characteristic of involving the redirection of attention from the sound of one's own voice on to that of the speaker who is being shadowed or monitored. Cherry and Sayers suggest that the well-documented observation that stutterers experience much reduced difficulty when speaking in chorus may well be an example of facility induced by the shadowing process.

Similarly, reading *simultaneously* from the same text with others who are fluent seems to have the effect of modifying and reducing stuttering. It is true that the stutterer may experience difficulty in initiating speech during the first few words of simultaneous reading (a factor which is discussed later in connection with the use of rhythm as an external control), but this difficulty soon passes and, typically, the stutterer can "settle down" to fluent speech in this situation.

At some stage it seems possible that changes can be introduced into either the shadowing or simultaneous speech situations, such as when the control subject switches to a different text to that being read by the stutterer, and this may take place without impairment of the latter's fluency. To Cherry and Sayers this suggests that it is the actual physical sounds made by the control speaker, rather than the specific words used, which effect the modification of speech abnormality. Switching to "gibberish", which has a similar phonetic structure to that of the language employed, is reported to be equally successful in inhibiting stuttering and consequently endorses the Cherry and Sayers hypothesis.

· Using such methods these investigators achieved a good measure of success in eliminating the speech abnormalities of stutterers, although they point out that individual differences are found in terms of speed of acquisition of the skill and the degree of efficiency attained.

These preliminary experiments suggested that the control is effected by acoustic elements through the mechanisms of *attention* rather than *meaning*.* However, it did not follow that all acoustic elements were involved, and it was therefore decided to investigate the respective influence of two fairly easily separable components—wave-conducted and bone-conducted sounds.

Two experiments were necessary to achieve this separation. In one, air-conducted sound was eliminated by blocking the ears of subjects, while in the other the elimination of both air- *and* bone-conducted sounds was accomplished by relaying a very loud masking noise through earphones.

The outcome of the first experiment showed very little or no effect upon stutters, but the conditions of the second experiment produced a virtual complete elimination of stuttering. This striking result

* In this connection it should be borne in mind that experimental evidence presented in Chapter 6 suggests that frequency of stuttering is related to the meaningfulness of words,

suggested to Cherry and Sayers that abnormalities of speech among stutterers might be related to D.A.F. through bone-conduction rather than air-conduction pathways. The results might indicate that, as there is some difference in the pitch of tones transmitted by these two pathways, the omission of low-frequency (bone-conducted) tones from speech could exercise considerable control of stuttering. This contention received support from further experiments which required normal subjects to experience purely bone-conducted delayed feedback through specially adapted electrical headphones attached to the temples, and also from other experiments in which subjects were asked to whisper. The former investigation produced the expected very marked impairment of fluency, while the latter (by cutting out low frequency tones) proved extremely effective in reducing stutters.

Cherry and Sayers agree that their procedures for effecting the modification and control of stutters could be considered to be part of a general class of techniques for *distracting* the stutterer. However, they claim that their analysis seems to point to the involvement of a more basic and important principle, and it must be conceded that an explanation in terms of a defect in auditory perception has greater incisiveness, generality, and explanatory power. One alternative explanation of their findings which they considered was that, as masking often induces people to speak more loudly, speaking loudly *alone* might effect some modification of speech disturbance. Accordingly an experiment was carried out in which subjects were required to speak quietly under the influence of masking, and the outcome enabled them to rule out the alternative hypothesis postulated.

In this connection it is interesting to speculate on the reasons for improvement in the fluency of stutterers when speaking loudly. It could be argued, from the explanatory model provided by Cherry and Sayers, that speaking loudly usually involves raising the pitch of the voice, and it may be that this to some extent eliminates the troublesome feedback of low frequency tones.

In further experiments along lines dictated by their preliminary inquiry, Cherry and Sayers used a masking white noise which could be relayed at either above or below 500 c/s. With the high frequency masking the speaker was only aware of his own low frequency tones, and stuttering remained severe; using a low frequency tone masking noise (i.e. cutting out perception of the speaker's own low frequency tones) produced the predicted increase in fluency. There was, however, variability of response to the latter condition, suggesting that the threshold of required modifying frequencies probably varies from one individual to another.

From their experiments with 54 stutterers these investigators felt able to conclude that stuttering is mediated by (if not *caused* by) a defect in the auditory perception of low frequency tones. Certainly a number of observations in the field of stuttering can be explained by adopting their hypothesis, among which is the finding reported by Harms and Malone (1939) that stuttering is extremely rare in the totally deaf.

There is still, however, the outstanding problem in D.A.F. work of why there are marked individual differences in response to this condition, with a few subjects showing little noticeable disturbance, most showing marked impairment, and a small proportion being totally incapacitated in their speech. To some extent verbal fluency appears to counteract D.A.F. effects (Arens and Popplestone, 1959), and there is some suggestion from the work of Spilka (1954) and Goldfarb and Braunstein (1958) that the degree of dependence upon internal and external cues is implicated. In both the latter studies the argument is indirect, involving the proposition that differential dependence upon these two types of cue is a function of personality characteristics. Both studies afford evidence of some relationship of the kind postulated, the latter study showing that while schizophrenic children were poorer under normal reading conditions they were, on average, superior to controls under conditions of D.A.F. These findings offer some tentative support for the explanation put forward by Cherry and Sayers, but it is unfortunate that the use of cues was not examined in a more direct way in these studies.

In this connection it might be noted that Goldiamond has observed that people who talk a great deal without apparently listening to themselves are less susceptible to D.A.F. influence. His notions in this respect are concerned with the degree of dependence upon feedback of auditory and proprioceptive cues in speech, and a fuller statement of his ideas is presented in a later section. However, it is sufficient here to point out that no solution to the problem of individual differences in reaction to D.A.F. has yet been presented. The answer to this question could have very important implications for any theory of perceptual defect in stutterers.

Another important aspect of the D.A.F. phenomenon and stuttering is that concerned with adaptation. Cherry and Sayers reported no tendency for adaptation to occur, but other studies suggest that this effect can occur to some degree. In one study, for example, Winchester *et al.* (1959) employed ten 200-syllable passages and found an increase in reading speed. In another study, by Tiffany and Hanley (1956), in which the subjects read a passage of prose twelve times on each of two occasions (the occasions being separated by a 1-week interval), it was found that fluency improved for the second set of trials. The effects of long-term practice with D.A.F. are not fully known but these results may suggest that adaptation effects could be present to an extent which might have allowed stutterers to compensate for any feedback delay, should this be their characteristic difficulty. However, the Cherry and Sayers findings have been independently investigated and endorsed by both Shane (1955) and by Maraist and Hutton (1957). In Shane's experiment masking noises of 95 db and 25 db were used as well as a "no noise" condition, the results indicating that the 95 db noise was highly effective while that of 25 db yielded no better results than the "no noise" condition.

On the other hand, noise volume may be found to be functionally related to stuttering modification. In the Maraist and Hutton study, for example, it was shown that a 90 db masking noise produced almost normal fluency and rate of reading in stutterers, but it also seemed that a 50 db white noise was sufficiently effective in reducing nonfluency to be clinically useful. This investigation, involving the testing of 15 adult stutterers under various levels of masking, showed that errors made per minute fell from an average of 26 without masking, to 6 with the 90 db noise. For the 30, 50, and 70 db noise levels stuttering errors were, on average, 22, 18, and 11 respectively.

One of the important questions bearing upon problems of D.A.F. and stuttering is that of whether the abnormalities of speech produced by D.A.F. in normals are like those found among stutterers under non-D.A.F. conditions. Using 23 stutterers, and the same number of non-stuttering controls, Neelley (1961) investigated the outcome of reading a 100-word passage on five separate occasions under non-D.A.F. conditions, and then under D.A.F. conditions 1 day later. He reported that the adaptation effect (i.e. the tendency for nonfluencies to diminish) among stutterers was different in both degree and kind from that found among normals reading under feedback delay of 0·14 second. Perhaps even more significant, however, was his finding that listeners had little difficulty in distinguishing the D.A.F. speech of normals from the speech of stutterers not influenced by D.A.F. conditions. Furthermore, listeners could not distinguish the speech of the two groups when both spoke under D.A.F. conditions. Neelley concluded that the evidence strongly indicated that the speech characteristics induced in normals by D.A.F. are quite different from those which are usually referred to as stuttering, and that the auditory feedback mechanism does not provide a satisfactory account of stuttering.

However, as Yates points out in his review paper (1963), Neelley's findings are based upon only one delay interval (0·14 second), and also that the normal subjects had clearly had much less practice in reading under D.A.F. conditions than the stutterers had of reading under normal conditions. It is generally agreed that the manifestations of stuttering undergo profound modifications and changes with the passing of time and it might be unreasonable to expect exactly the same type of nonfluency to emerge as that produced by D.A.F.

A further difficulty in interpretation of D.A.F. and masking is raised by Sutton and Chase in their paper (1961). They state that during the course of carrying out experiments using a variety of acoustic conditions in an effort to control stuttering, it seemed unlikely that "noise" produces its effect by preventing the stutterer from hearing the sound of his own voice. Accordingly an experiment was conducted in which five conditions were compared for their effect upon nine stutterers. The conditions were as follows: masking noise presented during phonation only, i.e. only when speech was produced; masking noise only during the silent periods *between* utterances; continuous masking throughout both speech and silent periods; wearing earphones alone without the presence of masking noise; a control condition without earphones or masking. It was evident from the results of this study that all the "noise" conditions were superior to "no noise" conditions respecting reduction of nonfluencies. However, no differences *between* the noise conditions were evident, suggesting that noise may not exert its influence through "drowning" the speaker's perception of his own voice. Sutton concludes that the mechanisms previously postulated as responsible for masking effects require reappraisal and that, in particular, the notion that noise is successful only in so far as it "blocks" the sound of the speaker's voice is possibly erroneous.

However, no straightforward interpretation of these results is possible. It may be, as Andrews and Harris (1964) suggest in connection with syllable-timed speech, that the separation of speech sounds into discrete units with small silences between them may offset the effects of "auditory lag" in stutterers. Noise may, under the conditions used by Sutton, simply have effected this kind of compensation.

In connection with the effects of D.A.F. upon speech, and the implications which this might have for stuttering, a study by Bachrach (1964) is of obvious interest. He appears to accept the contention that self-monitoring of speech is clearly related to stuttering, but feels it important to relate the effects of D.A.F. to the well-documented sex differences in frequency of stuttering. In other words, if stuttering is related to aspects of the feedback mechanisms, and stuttering is more pronounced among males, then one might reasonably expect a differential response by males and females to D.A.F. conditions.

Using eight male and eight female subjects and two conditions, masking by means of white noise, and D.A.F. (with a delay of $0 \cdot 2$–$0 \cdot 8$ second), Bachrach concluded that the results of his experiment were consistent both with the greater preponderance of stuttering among males and the proposition that the sexes appear to employ different "coping mechanisms". In particular, while varying degrees of artificial "stuttering" could be induced in males, no signs of "stuttering" were observed among the females. Also, deceleration of rate and decrease in intensity of speech were common in the former group, while the opposite effects seemed to be produced in the latter.

This experiment carries important implications for theories of D.A.F. and stuttering. Bachrach's idea of different "coping mechanisms" is too vague to be of much value, although differences between males and females in the use of perceptual cues has been noted in other connections. It may be that a much simpler explanation could fit Bachrach's findings as well as the explanatory principles put forward by Cherry and Sayers; for example it is possible that the voices of women are less likely to be characterized by a preponderance of low frequency tones.

In summary it might be said that experiments in D.A.F. and masking have advanced knowledge concerning their specific effects upon speech to a considerable extent but, as in any field of thriving research, discrepancies occur and these require explanation. However, it is fortunately often the case that in accounting for findings which are apparently at variance we are able to provide the answers to many important problems, and discrepancies are not always to be viewed with pessimism.

3. *Experimental Studies of the "Rhythm Effect"*

The use of rhythmical stimulation in the control of stuttering has enjoyed a very long history, probably extending over many centuries. By the nineteenth century the employment of rhythm as a main part of the therapeutic procedure for stuttering was well established, and in 1837 Serre d'Alais had introduced his "isochrome" (the forerunner of the metronome), whose beat was "followed" by the stutterer. Basically the same instrument made its appearance in the speech clinics of America under the new name of "orthophone", but subsequently the popularity of this "rhythm method" as a therapeutic tool rapidly declined.

Three main reasons seem to have been responsible for abandonment of rhythm in therapy; first, no obvious satisfactory explanation for its effectiveness could be given; secondly, that some degree of prejudice was aroused by the almost magical influence of a little-understood device which did not require the therapist to employ his skills; and thirdly, it was suggested that while the immediate results of the "rhythm effect" were good, the susceptibility to this form of control disappeared within a short time.

It is perhaps surprising that serious attempts to understand the mechanisms involved in the rhythm effect have been lacking. It may not be an exaggeration to say that an explanation of this most powerful influence upon stuttering should inevitably lead to a better understanding of the mechanisms of the disorder itself, and perhaps lead to a more effective form of therapy than any which is currently available. Such explanations as have been offered largely arise out of investigations, and accounts given, of other phenomena, rather than as the outcome of direct experimental attack upon the rhythm effect itself.

One kind of explanation which has been offered in this connection argues that, for some unspecified reason, the stutterer has some degree of inferiority or disability in the performance of motor skills. In this case externally imposed rhythm, for example by means of a metronome, is seen as affording compensation for the defect.

An early study with this orientation was reported by Blackburn (1931) who stated that stutterers were characterized by a marked inferiority to nonstutterers in the execution of voluntary tongue and diaphragm movements. He found that the difference between the groups did not, however, extend to movements other than those involved in speech. This is not altogether surprising. However, other studies were carried out which involved a measure of support for Blackburn's finding. Ingebregsten (1936), for example, reported that more than 40% of his sample of stutterers were unable to reproduce a melody and seemed to have little sense of rhythm, and Bilto's (1941) observations led him to conclude that children suffering from speech defects were inferior to a group of unimpaired children in rhythmical tasks, in co-ordination, and in strength.

A few years earlier, Bills (1934) had reported an interesting investigation in which he suggested that stuttering could be viewed as a form of blocking which could be observed in normal subjects. In support of a general characteristic of "blocking" he reported significant relationships (0·63 and 0·72) between manual and vocal blocks in terms of both their length and frequency. Comparing normals and stutterers on his measures he discovered that both manual as well as vocal blocks were longer and more frequent among the latter.

On the other hand there is, perhaps, a greater weight of evidence against the proposition that stutterers are inferior to nonstutterers in their appreciation and execution of rhythmical tasks. One such study has, for example, been conducted by Cross (1936) who found no differences between the two groups in terms of their motor capacities. In another investigation Rotter (1955) was unable to demonstrate differences between stutterers and nonstutterers in terms of their capacity for rhythmic co-ordination, and Ross (1955) could find no evidence for difference between the groups in respect of their performance on psychomotor tasks. Again, in two studies conducted by Strother and Kriegman (1943, 1944), no support was found for the existence of arrhythmokinesis in stutterers, and no differences were observed between this group and a group of controls in terms of rate of diadochokinetic movements of lips, mandible, tongue, or fingers.

The most popular alternative model put forward to account for the "rhythm effect" has been based upon the idea that rhythm acts as a distractor. This notion certainly has the advantage of fitting in quite well with the explanatory frameworks advocated to account for other stuttering phenomena. For example, it can be used as a common explanation to account for the success of masking effects (i.e. by reducing or eliminating the degree of attention paid by the stutterer to the sound of his own voice). By the same token, it could be argued that any theory dependent upon an anxiety reduction model could subsume the rhythm effect under the general category of conditions which lower the anxiety which may be induced by communicative responsibility.

The notion of the distractor in this connection has a ready appeal, for as Fletcher (1928) points out a wide variety of "therapeutic expedients" such as placing a cork between the teeth, shrugging the shoulders, speaking in an assumed voice, tapping the feet, whistling and counting before speaking, all seem to be at least temporarily effective. In these cases the general argument seems to be that the stutterer is bound up in his difficulty and concentrates his attentions and energies upon an activity (speaking) which is actually handicapped by this too-close conscious control. Diverting the attention achieves the effect of removing the speaker's "morbid" concentration from the activity of speech.

One of the more important early experimental investigations of the "rhythm effect" was that carried out on 18 stutterers by Johnson and Rosen (1937). The subjects in this study were required to read passages under a number of different conditions including variable speed, intensity, and pitch of speech, chorus reading, and differing "rhythm" conditions. It was found that all the imposed speech patterns constituting the "conditions" served to reduce the amount of stuttering, with the exception of "fast reading" which actually served to increase the number of nonfluencies. Of the methods which were effective, however, the imposition of rhythmical speech was stated to be the most efficient in reducing stutters. For example, the "rhythm effect" produced from one to eight speech errors in contrast to the 120 errors which occurred under conditions which simply involved a reduced rate of speech.

The design of this study unfortunately did not take account of adaptation effects (which can produce up to 50 % reduction in stuttering), and a direct comparison of speech errors produced under the various conditions could be misleading. However, the "rhythm effect" as assessed in this investigation was so powerful and compelling as to make perfect control for adaptation unnecessary to the conclusion that rhythm was superior to all other conditions employed.

Quite properly the authors point out that the use of the term "distraction" to account for the effects of rhythm lacks precision, and offer a more precise formulation in terms of variability in the degree of "stuttering expectancy" as being more satisfying. In other words it is postulated that under conditions of altered patterning of speech the stutterer is distracted from his tendency to *expect* stuttering to occur. While this notion does introduce some degree of refinement into the use of "distraction" in connection with nonfluencies of speech, it does not appear to be a fully acceptable account of why rhythm serves as a better distractor than any of the other methods employed in the experiment.

Relevant in this connection is a study by Barber (1939) who investigated the use of chorus reading as a "distractor". She felt able to rule out the possibility that stuttering was a phonetic disturbance, and postulated that the explanation for the decrement in stuttering found in chorus reading was that the speaker receives "support" from others. Reading without such "support" is seen as throwing a compelling responsibility upon the stutterer to speak well, and the greater the importance he attaches to this responsibility the more likely he will be to stutter.

Pattie and Knight (1944), on the other hand, also investigated the effects of chorus reading by comparing the performance of stutterers under various conditions. One of these involved the subject reading alone with no-one else present, another required the subject to read in unison with a fluent person in the same room. In a third condition reading in unison was carried out over a telephone, and in a fourth condition the subject read alone to an audience of three persons present in the same room. The number of "blocks" experienced under these conditions and others were compared, and it was found that while simultaneous reading produced from 14 to 23 "blocks" on average, the means experienced in other conditions ranged from 65 to 134. However, it was felt that the results were not consistent with Barber's contention that chorus reading is effective because the burden of communication is shared. Instead, Pattie and Knight argue that their results are more in line with the notion of chorus reading acting as a "pacemaker", by which they meant that the regular rhythmic cadence necessary to achieve synchrony in chorus reading operates like the metronome.

Barber (1940) has also reported a further experimental investigation of the effectiveness of rhythm in the control of stuttering. An interesting feature of this study was that the influence of rhythmic stimulation through three modalities (visual, auditory, and tactual) was observed. The results indicated that the influence of rhythm was equally effective whichever modality was involved, but it was also expected that there would be some interaction with speed of speech. This latter expectation was confirmed; using a metronomic rate of 184 beats per minute (b.p.m.) produced significantly greater amounts of stuttering than a rate of 92 b.p.m.

Further support for Barber's finding that the modality involved in the "rhythm effect" does not affect the total amount of stuttering produced, comes from a study by Meyer and Mair (1963). However, an interesting feature of Barber's results concerns the consistency of the control effected by different modality conditions for, in general, there seemed to be only a low or nonsignificant relationship between the amounts of stuttering which individuals produced under the various procedures employed. While the Meyer and Mair study also concluded that rhythmical stimulation in modalities other than auditory might be equally effective, it would seem that Barber's results suggest some degree of specificity in the modality control of stuttering.

The Meyer and Mair experiment (1963) is of particular value in assessing the clinical importance of the rhythm effect in the treatment of stuttering. Having no doubts concerning the degree of control exerted by using rhythmical speech, especially when a metronome is being "paced", these investigators were responsible for the construction of a device similar to a hearing aid which was capable of emitting a regular rhythmic beat. This instrument is essentially portable and should cause little embarrassment as the beats would ordinarily not be audible to anyone but the wearer.

The authors report the results of using this apparatus (AP) on five stutterers, all but one of whom had previously received treatment which had been unsuccessful (e.g. speech therapy, hypnosis, shadowing, and psychotherapy). Patients were first instructed to wear the AP in all situations and to speak "with the rhythm" until they achieved some degree of fluency in a situation. At this stage the patient was asked to switch off the AP but continue to speak "as if the rhythm were still present". However, should he meet or anticipate difficulty then he should switch on the AP once again. When fluency had been achieved to a large extent the patient was asked to dispense with the AP altogether. This gradual weaning of dependency upon AP was matched by the provision of graded tasks in which the patient first engaged in those situations which were less productive of stutters, and only later encountered those conditions which, prior to AP training, produced the most severe forms of nonfluency.

The results, from the standpoint of therapy, were mixed. While all five patients showed initial improvement, the tendency to relapse after gaining a reasonable degree of fluency seemed to be a very real possibility. Why the relapses should occur on occasion has considerable interest for both theorists and practitioners. There could be one of at least two possible explanations; either the psychological "gain" from fluency is less than satisfying to the stutterer, or that through some process of "adaptation" the rhythm ceases to exercise its former function. What this function is, of course, has not as yet been determined, but Meyer and Mair quote an additional investigation on two subjects which attempts to deal with and analyse the possible components of the rhythm effect.

Briefly, this additional investigation suggested that while regular rhythm of 90 b.p.m. produced complete fluency, faster regular beats and irregular but predictable rhythms were less effective, while irregular and unpredictable beats did not seem to modify stuttering at all. They conclude that these findings suggest that the "rhythm effect" does not depend simply upon a kind of distraction.

This conclusion was also drawn by Beech and Debbane (1962) in an independent investigation of a single case. The hypotheses tested were, first that rhythm usually exerts its influence on stuttering by slowing down the rate of speech; typically stutterers are described as rushing headlong into speech, and it seemed possible that this alone could be productive of nonfluency. Secondly, it was hypothesized that rhythm may simply serve to distract the stutterer and that any other form of distracting stimulus, for example an irregular as opposed to a regular tone, would be equally effective. Neither hypothesis was confirmed in this study although for methodological considerations it seemed desirable to repeat the investigation using larger numbers and more careful controls.

Accordingly a further study was carried out by Fransella and Beech (1965) with the specific aims of demonstrating the extent of control achieved by rhythmic speech, testing the hypothesis that rhythm exerts its influence by operating as a "distractor", and examining the proposition that the effect can be obtained by regulating the speed of speech of the stutterer. In this experiment, involving eighteen male stutterers, three experimental conditions were employed, "rhythmic metronome", "arrhythmic metronome", and "no metronome", each condition being administered under "usual" and "slow" rates of speech. In this connection it might be pointed out that Fransella devised a method of predicting the stutterer's "usual" rate of speech, independent of stutters, by examining the relationship between the "silent" and "aloud" reading rates of normals.

The results of their experiment clearly indicated the success of the rhythmic metronome condition as shown in Fig. 23, and this condition was significantly differentiated from the other two in terms of speech errors produced. On the other hand, the "arrhythmic" and "no metronome" conditions were not differentiated at an acceptable level of significance. It was concluded that this evidence strongly suggested that the "rhythm effect" is *not* achieved because it functions as a

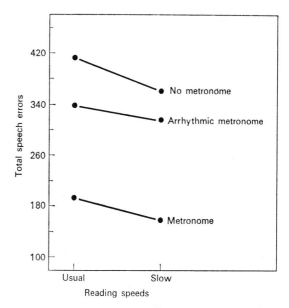

FIG. 23. Total speech errors elicited at "usual" and "slow" speeds by the three metronome conditions in group rhythm experiment (Fransella, 1965a).

"distractor" in a simple and obvious sense, especially as the instructions in the "arrhythmic" condition required subjects to pay careful attention to the beats in order to detect any patterning. (The beats in this condition were, in fact, random.)

Summing the results of all three conditions it was found that the "speed" factor was significant, the slower rate producing fewer errors overall, and that this effect was *independent* of the "rhythm effect". It appeared to be the case that speed of speech exerted a significant but less important influence than rhythm upon the number of nonfluencies produced, but that, as these two influences are not intercorrelated, rhythm does not derive its particular power from any reduction in the speed of speech which might be involved. Indeed, as the predicted "usual speed of speech" for stutterers was, if anything, slower than that of normals, the hypothesis that stutterers "rush" their speech seems to have been unlikely in the first place.

However, Fransella (1967) thought it still possible that the arrhythmic beat had failed to effect a significant decrease in stuttering because it did not demand the continuous attention of the stutterer. Certainly it is possible to argue that with a rhythmic beat the stutterer is an active participant in a different sense than that which might describe his activities in speaking in the presence of an arrhythmic stimulus. This proposition was tested by comparing the errors made under the standard "rhythmic metronome" condition with those occurring when reading and at the same time performing a subsidiary task. In this experiment the subsidiary task involved writing down a continuous series of numbers relayed by a tape recorder.

The outcome was clear-cut. The average number of errors produced under the standard metronome condition was 5·17, while that for the subsidiary task condition was 13·56, and this highly significant difference again casts doubt on the proposition that the "rhythm effect" derives its influence from its capacity to distract. This conclusion is further endorsed by the finding that no significant difference in fluency existed between the subsidiary task condition and a control ("no task, no rhythm") condition.

While alternative explanations for these results cannot be ruled out (e.g. insufficient distraction, too much distraction, heightened anxiety being involved in the "distraction" conditions), several tentative conclusions might be drawn at this stage. First, that the rhythm effect is a powerful means of modifying stuttering behaviour; secondly, that it is not dependent for its effect upon any tendency to reduce the speed of speech; and thirdly, that there is no evidence that distraction, as measured, effects any modification of nonfluencies.

These results tell us what the rhythm effect does *not* do, but they fail to inform us as to the particular mechanisms through which this influence *does* operate so successfully.

However, Beech and Fransella (1966) have undertaken a further study in which the proposition is tested that rhythm is effective by virtue of its capacity to make *essentially predictable* the point in time at which vocalization should occur. Should this explanation be correct, then other techniques which provide cues defining the time at which speech should be initiated, other than those involving the superimposition of rhythm on speech, should be equally successful in the modification of stuttering. The central idea in this proposition is quite consistent with findings reported by Brown (1938), namely that more than 90% of stutters occur in relation to the initial sounds of words, and that more stuttering is evident for *first* words of sentences and paragraphs than for any other word position.

Twenty stutterers served as their own controls in the experiment which involved a comparison of the difficulty experienced in reading words which were exposed on a screen for varying lengths of time. For half the words used the point in time at which they were to be pronounced was clearly indicated, while for the other words the utterance was required at unspecified moments during their exposure.

The results confirmed the hypothesis, indicating that some means of enabling subjects to determine the moment at which an utterance should occur serves to facilitate fluency. However, the effect in terms of the present results, while highly significant, did not appear to be sufficiently powerful to account for all the corrective influence exerted by rhythm.

Finally, in this section concerning the control of stuttering through the "rhythm principle", mention should be made of a study reported by Andrews and Harris (1964). Altogether 35 subjects were used, 5 being school-children and the remainder ranging in age from 16 to 45 years, and all were taught to use syllable-timed speech (ST-speech). This method involves the removal of all stress and syllable contrasts, each syllable being pronounced and stressed evenly and rhythmically. Most subjects received about 100 hours of practice, beginning with simple sentences repeated after the therapist, and later with spontaneous conversations as speed and fluency of speech improved.

Subjects were reviewed regularly for periods ranging from 6 months to 1 year.

Prior to treatment the subjects, who had been split into four groups, had experienced an average rate of stutter of 20 in every 100 words. Following the intensive course in ST-speech, very great improvement was noted in all groups, and the group ratings employed by Andrews and Harris suggested that the shift had been from "severe" to "mild" degree of stutter as characteristic of the groups as a whole.

At the 3-month check, however, relapse had occurred in all groups, although the average severity of stutter at this time was not quite as great as that found prior to commencement of treatment. Follow-up at the end of a 12-month period indicated that no general shift had occurred during the period following the 3-month check.

It is of interest to note that while the two adult groups and the adolescent group appeared to fare as well or as badly as each other, the group of children did significantly better in that their degree of improvement attributed to ST-speech was greater. The children actually did show exactly the same trend for relapse to occur, but here the relapse was not total and a greater degree of improvement was maintained by the group members than was the case for the adults and adolescents. These differential results obtained for children are tentatively explained as being attributable to the earlier stage of the disorder which they had reached before treatment began (i.e. there were fewer "secondary complications" such as grimacing), and also because they were not generally as emotionally disturbed as were some of the older subjects.

While regarding the method of ST-speech as being simply part of the general class of rhythm control agents, Andrews and Harris briefly speculate about the possible mechanisms involved. They suggest that as it might be possible that stutterers experience delay in the feedback of speech, it could be that leaving an interval of silence between speaking syllables has the advantage of allowing accurate perception to occur before the next syllable is attempted. However, they point out that even if evidence could be collected in support of this hypothesis, one would still be left with the problem of explaining how it is that reinstatement of normal speech, at least temporarily, is possible by utilizing ST-methods, i.e. how do stutterers achieve speech which is not punctuated by silent intervals?

Research into the rhythm effect has not so far produced more than a tantalizing glimpse of the mechanisms which may be involved. Clearly no satisfactory explanation has been found so far for the surprisingly efficient control which this technique affords. There also remains some doubt concerning the lasting effects of rhythm training and perhaps, from a therapeutic standpoint, this is one of the most pressing considerations.

STUDIES IN THE MODIFICATION OF STUTTERING

4. *Operant Conditioning and Stuttering*

The central proposition or principle involved in operant conditioning is that the consequences which follow a particular piece of behaviour influence the future occurrence of that behaviour. Consequences which are usually referred to as "rewards" are, of course, most commonly observed to be associated with increased frequency in the behaviour which precedes them.

Thorndike is usually credited with having put forward the first systematic exposition of this principle, but his account in terms of the strengthening of behaviour which had "satisfying" consequences and the weakening of behaviour which resulted in "dissatisfying" consequences, is limited. Skinner and his associates have, on the other hand, been mainly responsible for elucidating the principle in greater detail and demonstrating its application to simple and complex behaviour in humans and other species, and have also developed a number of ingenious experiments in which operant conditioning has been studied. While it is the case that the psychological bases of the reinforcement principle are not fully understood, the principle itself may still be useful as, from it, behaviour can be predicted and controlled, sometimes with great precision.

It is obvious that rewards, or positive reinforcers, serve to strengthen behaviour; this is a matter of common observation which detailed experimentation serves to refine. Less well understood is the action of negative reinforcers, and these are *not* usually best defined as stimuli which produce decrement in the frequency of a particular piece of behaviour; quite often such stimuli serve to *strengthen* that behaviour, for example behaviour which leads to the removal of painful effects. The strengthening of a response through negative reinforcement is illustrated by the kind of experiment in which the rat escapes the effects of an electric shock by pressing a lever, and "bar pressing" under these conditions is quickly learned and retained.

However, the negative reinforcer may also have the function of *reducing* the occurrence of some aspect of behaviour. In this context the negative reinforcer is often referred to as an "aversive stimulus" and defines those situations where such a stimulus *follows* the behaviour in question.

We have, therefore, two kinds of outcome depending upon the mode of action of the negative reinforcement. In one, the behaviour serves to remove the stimulus and is strengthened as a result; in the other the negative reinforcement follows the behaviour and, as a result, weakens the tendency for that behaviour to occur on future occasions. As will be shown later in this section, both "escape" and "punishment" have been studied by Goldiamond in relation to stuttering.

These principles are relatively easy to understand and to demonstrate; the difficult task, which has been the main concern of Skinner and others, is that of investigating the variables which determine the particular outcome of attempts to apply the principles in practice. For example, studies have been carried out concerning the specific operation of various types and schedules of reinforcement as well as of the various intervals which may separate the stimulus and the response.

Of special interest to those involved in the field of stuttering and operant procedures, and the important variables associated with the latter, is the area of verbal conditioning.

This term refers to the application of positive and negative reinforcements to particular types and classes of verbalization with the aim of influencing the output of this form of behaviour.

Much evidence has now accumulated showing that verbal behaviour can be modified and changed by operant conditioning principles, and useful summaries of this evidence have been provided by Krasner (1958) and Greenspoon (1962). While it is the case that there are sometimes reports of negative results, i.e. where there has been failure to secure satisfactory evidence for conditioning, it seems likely that to some extent the many powerful influences involved in complex verbal situations might be responsible. For example, Greenspoon (1962) has reported finding that increments in the use of plural nouns through positive reinforcement was more difficult to obtain than in the case of non-plural nouns, and a study by Ball (1953) suggests that the type of positive reinforcer offered has a significant influence upon response rate. Also implicated are the characteristics of the subject, the person administering reinforcement, anxiety, as well as numerous other variables.

It would be of considerable interest to apply the findings from the field of verbal conditioning to the special area of stuttering. Certainly the evidence for regarding verbal behaviour as susceptible to operant procedures is quite compelling, and it is not surprising that interest has been aroused in applying such procedures to stuttering. So far,

relatively little work has been done in this respect beyond the collection
of some preliminary results which suggest that stuttering can be considered as an example of operant behaviour, and that the possibility
of using operant methods for the control of this disorder holds
considerable promise.

There is general agreement on the question of nonfluencies in the
early years of life of the young child; at this stage repetitions,
prolongations, and other speech "difficulties" occur frequently and
can be said to have a high operant level. In addition, it has been
suggested (Davis, 1939, 1940a, b) that certain common types of
nonfluency in young children are concerned with securing attention,
seeking status, acquisition tendencies, criticizing, etc., so that these
phenomena of speech tend to be associated with situations in which
the speaker is manipulating the listener. The possibility therefore
exists that the response made by the listener to the speaker could
come to exercise some control over the latter's verbal behaviour.

In an interesting paper Shames and Sherrick (1963) set out the
case for regarding stuttering as a form of operant behaviour, and a
summary of their argument forms a useful introduction to work in
this topic area. They begin by pointing out that the behaviour of
parents in response to the child's "manding" behaviour is usually
unsystematic and unlike the strict schedules of reinforcement which
can be arranged in the psychological laboratory. However, if, for
example, speech repetitions are at all frequently related to variations
in reinforcement afforded by the parent, then this form of nonfluency
should appear in greater strength. An example of what might happen
is that a parent may delay reinforcement of the child's first verbalization, and the child is then led to repeat the utterance several times.
After several repetitions the parent may provide the positive reinforcement which the child demanded, perhaps being unaware that
he is rewarding speech repetition, and thus rendering such behaviour
more likely to occur again. Shames and Sherrick point out that this
situation, in their opinion, can often be found in the developmental
history of the stutterer. Perhaps the parent for some reason cannot
provide immediate reinforcement, thus encouraging verbal repetitions
by the child, which are eventually reinforced. The recurrence of
the rewarded repetitive verbalization is, however, annoying and the
parent may now resort to punishment in an attempt to terminate the
child's "nagging". However, discriminations will be made by
the child between situations where repetitions *are* reinforced and

those where a single utterance is sufficient to secure satisfactory responses.

Repetition may also occur in particular circumstances which are characterized by strong aversive elements. Here the repetitive behaviour may assume an avoidance character, i.e. it might serve to delay or avoid the aversive implications of the full and complete utterance as, for example, in confessing a mistake.

They may also occur in connection with certain conventions of speech, one of the "rules" of which is that "polite conversation" requires sharing of "speech time"; silence of one speaker is the cue for the listener to assume the role of speaker. Sometimes, however, the silence may not be a cue for speech by the second person, and any attempt to speak at this time may lead to interruption (perhaps with annoyance) by the first speaker who resumes verbalization. It is argued that, should this happen frequently, then the second speaker may develop a pattern of speech characterized by repetitions and long silences. Under these circumstances a child may emit the first sound in a silent period and wait to see if an interruption occurs, i.e. he *tests out* the situation to see whether or not it is a silence which invites speech on his part. Should the interruption *not* arrive then the child can continue by repeating his first utterance after a brief pause.

Shames and Sherrick also point out that during the act of communication "composition" often takes place as verbalization continues. This activity of "composing" is marked by hesitations, repetitions, and corrections to what has been said, and these modifications to on-going speech are capable of providing both positive and negative self-reinforcements for the speaker. Under these circumstances repetitions may serve the function of keeping the attention of the listener and also of filling the silent periods during "composition", so that "listener interruption" is made less likely.

In essence this view of stuttering as operant behaviour involves three basic propositions:

1. That there is some continuity between nonfluency in the child and the development of stuttering, i.e. it is possible to see how certain aspects of a child's utterances are related to stuttering.
2. That the environmental circumstances associated with the particular forms, changes, developments and modifications of nonfluency can be identified and described.
3. That the schedules and kinds of reinforcement involved in the

development and maintenance of stuttering are probably numerous and complex, i.e. there is probably no one single contingency for stuttering.

In their paper Shames and Sherrick not only provide a basis in theory for regarding stuttering as a form of operant behaviour, but also outline a case for the kind of experimentation which would be necessary to the development and testing of their position.

Goldiamond (1965), however, has been mainly responsible for the impetus given to operant analysis of stuttering behaviour. The position which he adopts is that stuttering can be defined as the high rate of occurrence of certain forms of speech (repetitions, hesitations, etc.), and that these characteristics occur so infrequently in normal speech that no problem is apparent. Continuity between "normal" and "stuttered" speech is therefore proposed, with frequency of occurrence postulated as the distinguishing feature.

In a first experiment by Flanagan et al. (1958), subjects were asked to read aloud for 90 minutes. After 30 minutes one of two conditions was imposed, either simple recording of nonfluencies or application of an aversive stimulus (very loud white noise) immediately following a nonfluency.

The results of this experiment showed quite unequivocally that punishment (i.e. a noxious stimulus following an "error") was extremely effective in controlling nonfluencies. In one subject stuttering was almost entirely eliminated at the end of a 30-minute punishment period and, perhaps just as important, the effects on speech were maintained for a few minutes following cessation of punishment. There was, however, a subsequent fairly rapid tendency to revert to the stuttering rate characteristic of the pre-training period.

In a second experiment negative reinforcement in an *escape context* was employed, where stuttering was arranged to have the effect of switching off the noxious white noise. In this experiment the predicted *increase* in rate of stuttering was found.

These experiments, taken together, constitute a substantial case for the contention that stuttering is affected by its consequences, diminishing under aversive stimulus conditions and increasing under other appropriate conditions of negative reinforcement.

In a further study the lapses in fluency of a *normally fluent* subject were increased by employing escape conditions. Here the subject was given continuous shock which could be switched off whenever disfluency occurred and, by recycling, a sufficiently high rate of disfluency could lead to continued avoidance of shock.

The results of this experiment were of great interest not only in showing that speech difficulties of "normals" can be considerably increased by appropriate conditions (with all that this might imply for theories about "the stutterer"), but also in respect of finding that the disfluencies persisted over a lengthy period of time. This latter point might suggest that as the *absence* of shock (escape from shock) served to maintain disfluencies, so *cessation* of shock also continued to maintain this behaviour.

In further studies by Goldiamond long-term investigations (up to 9 months) were carried out on 5 stutterers, "running" these subjects for 90 minutes each day for 5 days every week. In these cases it was decided to use delayed auditory feedback as a consequence of stutters, primarily because loud noise and electric shock have less to recommend them in clinical practice. Here D.A.F. was either made *contingent* upon stuttering (i.e. punishment), its elimination was *achieved* by stuttering, it was simply presented continuously, or it was completely absent.

Punishment produced results similar to those obtained previously. For one subject, before punishment conditions were introduced, 5100 words were read and difficulty occurred in connection with more than half of them; when D.A.F. was made contingent upon stuttering, reading rate doubled and stuttering was cut to about 1500 words. The results of continuous D.A.F. conditions, on the other hand, did not appear to have the same moderating influence upon stutters, indicating that the D.A.F. needed to be *response contingent* to achieve its effect.

For another subject D.A.F. was played continuously but it was arranged that nonfluencies were able to "buy" normal feedback for periods of 10 seconds. This initially produced both a drop in reading and stuttering rates, although subsequently both showed marked increases. In other words the result was an *increase* in that behaviour (stuttering) which had the effect of eliminating D.A.F., indicating that D.A.F. was aversive. However, it seemed to Goldiamond that two alternating patterns of response were observable, one characterized by a high reading and stuttering rate, and the other by a low rate of reading and little nonfluency. This particular subject eventually "settled for" the latter pattern and this pattern persisted for some time even though negative reinforcement was discontinued.

However, for another subject, while the use of response contingent D.A.F. reduced stuttering rate, making elimination of D.A.F. contingent upon stuttering also had this effect. Clearly, if D.A.F. was aversive (as other data suggested) then the latter condition should have produced an increase rather than a decrease in stuttering rate. Accordingly an investigation of the effects of D.A.F. was conducted.

Goldiamond points out that auditory stimuli are contingent upon verbal behaviour and may serve to maintain it, in which case this "feedback" can be seen as reinfoicing. However, if the feedback is *delayed* (i.e. the reinforcement is deferred) this may have the effect of prolonging the speech behaviour so that response and reinforcement again are made immediately contingent. On the other hand, proprioceptive stimuli may also assume a reinforcing function in speech and would not, of course, be altered by delaying auditory feedback. Anyone dependent upon auditory feedback for reinforcement would suffer disruption of speech, but immediate reinstatement of reinforcement would be possible for the individual capable of switching from auditory to proprioceptive input. Accordingly, an experiment was carried out in which subjects were asked to listen to, or not to listen to, what they said under D.A.F. conditions, and the results were in line with Goldiamond's contention. This outcome suggests that differential dependence upon, or ability to switch dependence from, auditory and proprioceptive feedback could account for any conflicting results which might be obtained. From this point Goldiamond elected to investigate the outcome of using a particular programme of training. This involved first establishing a new verbal response pattern by securing the kind of D.A.F. prolongation of speech which emerged unsolicited from earlier studies. Secondly, methods were used to make this behaviour responsive to general conditions as well as to those specific to the laboratory setting. Thirdly, because the prolongation speech pattern is a peculiar one, a programme of "shaping" would be utilized to make the pattern like that of normal speech. Finally, training would be given to enable this new speech pattern to be utilized outside the laboratory setting.

The preliminary results on several subjects have been encouraging although incomplete. Laboratory stuttering is said to have been completely eliminated, and speech has been well articulated and at a reasonable rate. In certain cases this improvement has extended to situations outside the laboratory.

The procedure has now been refined by Goldiamond and his colleagues to the point where relatively short periods of time are involved in treatment.

A main criticism of this work which has been anticipated by Goldiamond is that stuttering may represent a means of manipulating the environment, and that removing this "symptom" might result in the development of others. Goldiamond quite rightly contends that this argument can only be resolved by considering the facts, and these are not at present available. On the other hand, he concedes that it is possible that some other maladaptive process may lie "behind" the stutter, but argues that even if this were the case symptomatic treatment could still be an effective means of effecting better all-round adjustment. This argument is a familiar one in the context of treatment of nocturnal enuresis by the bell-and-blanket method and the outcome here has suggested not only that symptom substitution does not occur, but also that certain behavioural difficulties associated with the disturbance tend to "evaporate" when bladder control has been established.

Only further research and experience will resolve this problem in relation to stuttering, but the studies so far conducted into the application of operant procedures to the control of nonfluencies hold considerable promise that stuttering might be reduced or eliminated without unfortunate consequences. However, certain other problems are raised by Goldiamond's work, especially in relation to punishment as a therapeutic aid.

In general, punishment for nonfluencies has been cited as both a cause of stuttering and as an influence which exacerbates the disorder. Usually the view is taken that punishment conditions serve to evoke anxiety, or to raise anxiety levels, to a point where there is active interference with the execution of a skilled response (speech). The operation of anxiety as a disruptive influence in the performance of complex responses is not a new idea and much evidence is available in the psychological literature to substantiate the relationship. In this connection two studies by Goss (1952, 1956) are of interest not only in suggesting that anxiety is related to stuttering behaviour, but also that the way in which this variable operates in relation to stuttering could be of therapeutic interest. Briefly, this evidence indicates that stuttering varies as a function of the interval separating the cue to say a word and the exposure of that word; Goss interprets this as an illustration of Mowrer's (1938, 1940) contention that temporal factors exert an important influence upon the strength of anxiety.

Certain studies, for example, that were carried out by Van Riper (1937) to study the effects of threatened electric shock on speech, and that by Hill (1954) who examined the effect of actual electric shock on fluency, suggest that speech errors are increased by those conditions. However, these studies did not involve the contingent relationship of shock and speech difficulty and other investigations point to different outcomes of associating shock with nonfluency.

These discrepant findings are probably more apparent than real and may stem largely from the different conditions employed in various experiments.

An attempt to clarify these issues was made by Siegel and Martin (1965a, b) using normal subjects. Four separate conditions were utilized; threatened shock (but none actually delivered), shock given contingent upon the production of a disfluency, randomly administered electric shock, and a "no-shock" control condition. Two main outcomes were noted. First, it was clear that fluency among the subjects was susceptible to experimental modification, and secondly that when electric shock was made contingent upon the production of disfluency the result was generally to produce a decrement in this type of response.

The results in respect of the "threatened shock" condition were more equivocal, for the general trend was toward a *reduction* in the frequency of disfluency. Random shock, on the other hand, was associated with an increase in the number of disfluencies produced.

The reduction in speech errors noted under operant conditions is at least partial confirmation of Goldiamond's findings and is satisfying in that sense. However, as Siegel and Martin point out, generalizations about the influence of punishment on the disfluencies of normally fluent persons (or of stutterers for that matter) should be made only when the relevant variables and conditions can be specified.

In a further experiment (1965b) Siegel and Martin investigated 40 non-stutterers in an attempt to replicate their previous findings respecting the effects of response-contingent and random punishment. In this study it was decided to utilize the verbal punishment of the word "wrong" as an alternative to electric shock. The results confirmed those of their previous study but in a more clear-cut way; response-contingent punishment produced a substantial decrease in disfluency while the removal of punishment effected a return to the previous operant level of speech errors. This time, no change in fluency was associated with the application of random punishment.

Finally, in this section, a recent study by Daly and Cooper is of interest. They point out that while certain studies have used electric shock applied *after* the stuttering act, it may make more sense to shock the stutterer *during* the nonfluent period. The former procedure may have, as its basis, the notion that anxiety reduction occurs when the stuttered word is finally pronounced, and here shock is being used to inhibit the "relief" so obtained. The latter procedure (that of administering shock *during* the stutter) makes use of the experimental escape paradigm and depends upon the argument that anxiety reduction is occurring *during* the act of stuttering, i.e. the escape act itself is the anxiety-reducing agent.

The experimental procedure involved having 18 stutterers read a prose passage 5 times in succession, with three conditions being employed—shock *following* each example of nonfluency, shock *during* a stuttered utterance, and a "no-shock" control condition.

The results, evaluated in terms of the effects upon the degree of adaptation observed during the experiment, were equivocal respecting the rival propositions examined. Both "shock" conditions produced significantly less stuttering than the "no-shock" condition, but the former were not differentiated and there were no observable effects of shock upon adaptation rate.

The idea that an operant framework can be applied to stuttering behaviour is comparatively recent, but sufficient work has already been carried out which endorses the value of this approach. It is abundantly evident also that the field of stuttering is rich in opportunity for the specialist in operant procedures and that benefits to operant research as well as to stuttering research are likely to accrue. There is also little doubt that this approach has the kind of refreshingly direct quality which could produce significant advances in the treatment of speech disturbance.

5. *Conclusions*

1. Investigations of delayed auditory feedback suggest the possibility of a perceptual defect in stutterers.

2. The findings concerning D.A.F. masking procedures, and "rhythm control" of stuttering, may be related in terms of common mechanisms.

3. Neither the "distraction" hypothesis nor the "speed of speech" hypothesis appear to account for the high degree of control over stuttering which is exerted during rhythmical speech.

4. The beneficial effects of "rhythm" training often appear to be short-lived.

5. Studies so far conducted suggest that stuttering can be viewed as "operant" behaviour, and can be successfully modified by the appropriate use of reinforcements.

REFERENCES

ABBOTT, J. (1947) Repressed hostility as a factor in adult stuttering. *J. Sp. Hear. Dis.* **12**, 428–30.

ABORN, M., RUBENSTEIN, H. and STERLING, T. D. (1959) Sources of contextual constraint upon words in sentences. *J. Exp. Psychol.* **57**, 171–80.

ADAMS, M. R. and DIETZE, D. A. (1965) A comparison of the reaction times of stutterers and nonstutterers to items on a word association test. *J. Sp. Hear. Res.* **8**, 195–202.

AINSWORTH, C. (1939) Studies in the psychology of stuttering. XII. Empathic breathing of auditors while listening to stuttering speech. *J. Sp. Dis.* **4**, 149–56.

ANASTASI, A. (1958) *Differential Psychology*, 3rd ed., McMillan, New York.

ANASTASI, A. (1961) *Psychological Testing*, 2nd ed., McMillan, New York.

ANDERSON, J. and WHEALDON, M. L. (1941) A study of the blood group distribution among stutterers. *J. Sp. Dis.* **6**, 23–28.

ANDREWS, G. and HARRIS, M. (1964) *The Syndrome of Stuttering*, the Spastics Society Medical Education and Information, Heinemann, London.

APPELT, A. (1911) *The Real Cause of Stammering and its Permanent Cure*, Methuen, London.

ARENS, C. J. and POPPLESTONE, J. A. (1959) Verbal facility and delayed speech feedback. *Perc. Mot. Skills* **9**, 270.

AREND, R., HANDZEL, L. and WEISS, B. (1962) Dysphatic stuttering. *Folia Phoniat.* **14**, 55.

ARTHURS, R. G. S., CAPPON, D., DOUGLASS, E. and QUARRINGTON, B. (1954) Carbon dioxide therapy for stutterers. *Dis. Nerv. System* **15**, 123–26.

BACHRACH, D. L. (1964) Sex differences in reactions to delayed auditory feedback. *Perc. Mot. Skills* **19**, 81–82.

BALL, R. S. (1953) Reinforcement conditioning of verbal behaviour by verbal and nonverbal stimuli in a situation resembling a clinical interview. Ph.D. diss. Indiana Univ.

BARBER, V. B. (1939) Studies in the psychology of stuttering. XV. Chorus reading as a distraction in stuttering. *J. Sp. Dis.* **4**, 371–83.

BARBER, V. B. (1940) Studies in the psychology of stuttering. XVI. Rhythm as a distraction in stuttering. *J. Sp. Dis.* **5**, 29–42.

BARR, H. (1940) A quantitative study of the specific phenomena observed in stuttering. *J. Sp. Dis.* **5**, 277–80.

BARRON, F. (1953) An ego-strength scale which predicts response to psychotherapy. *J. Consult. Psychol.* **17**, 327–33.

BEECH, H. R. and DEBBANE, J. (1962) Unpublished manuscript.

BEECH, H. R. and FRANSELLA, FAY (1966) Research into rhythm effects. *Proc. Internat. Seminar on Stuttering and Behaviour Therapy*, Carmel, California.

BELL, A. M. (1853) *Observations on Defects of Speech, the Cure of Stammering, and the Principals of Elocution*, London.

BENDER, J. (1935) What the physical education instructor can do for the stuttering student. *J. Health Physical Educ.* **6**, 16.

BENDER, J. (1942) The stuttering personality. *Am. J. Orthopsychiat.* **12**, 140–6.

BERGER, E. M. (1952) The relation between expressed acceptance of self and expressed acceptance of others. *J. Abn. Soc. Psychol.* **47**, 778–82.

BERLIN, C. I. (1960) Parents' diagnoses of stuttering. *J. Sp. Hear. Res.* **3**, 372–9.

BERRY, M. F. (1932) A study of the medical histories of stuttering children. *Sp. Monogr.* **5**, 97–114.

BERRY, M. F. (1938) A common denominator in twinning and stuttering. *J. Sp. Hear. Dis.* **3**, 51–57.

BERRY, M. F. and EISENSON, J. (1956) *Speech Disorders: Principles and Practices of Therapy*, Appleton, New York.

BERWICK, NAOMI (1955) Stuttering in response to photographs of selected listeners. In *Stuttering in Children and Adults*, ed. W. Johnson, Univ. Minnesota Press, Minneapolis.

BILLS, A. G. (1934) The relation of stuttering to mental fatigue. *J. Exp. Psychol.* **17**, 574–84.

BILTO, E. W. (1941) A comparative study of certain physical abilities of children with speech defects and children with normal speech. *J. Sp. Dis.* **6**, 187–203.

BLACKBURN, W. B. (1931) Study of voluntary movements in stutterers and normal speakers. *Psychol. Monogr.* **41**, 1–13.

BLOODSTEIN, O. (1944) Studies in the psychology of stuttering. XIX. The relationship between oral reading and severity of stuttering. *J. Sp. Dis.* **9**, 161–73.

BLOODSTEIN, O. (1960a) The development of stuttering. I. Changes in nine basic features. *J. Sp. Hear. Dis.* **25**, 219–37.

BLOODSTEIN, O. (1960b) The development of stuttering. II. Developmental phases. *J. Sp. Hear. Dis.* **25**, 366–76.

BLOODSTEIN, O. (1961) The development of stuttering. III. Theoretical and clinical implications. *J. Sp. Hear. Dis.* **26**, 67–81.

BLOODSTEIN, O., JAEGER, W. and TUREEN, J. (1952) A study of the diagnosis of stuttering by parents of stutterers and nonstutterers. *J. Sp. Hear. Dis.* **17**, 308–15.

BLOODSTEIN, O. and SCHRIEBER, L. R. (1957) Obsessive–compulsive reactions in stutterers. *J. Sp. Hear. Dis.* **22**, 31–39.

BLOODSTEIN, O. and SMITH, S. (1954) A study of the diagnosis of stuttering with special reference to the sex ratio. *J. Sp. Hear. Dis.* **19**, 459–66.

BLUEMEL, C. S. (1957) *The Riddle of Stuttering*, the Instate Publishing Co., Danville, U.S.A.

BOEHMLER, R. M. (1958) Listener responses to nonfluencies. *J. Sp. Hear. Res.* **1**, 132–41.

BOLAND, J. L. JR. (1952) A comparison of stutterers and nonstutterers on several measures of anxiety. Ph.D. thesis, Univ. Michigan.

BRANCH, C., MILNER, B. and RASMUSSEN, T. (1964) Intracarotid sodium amytal for the lateralization of cerebral speech dominance observations in 123 patients. *J. Neurosurg.* **21**, 399–405.

BROWN, S. F. (1937) The influence of grammatical function on the incidence of stuttering. *J. Sp. Dis.* **2**, 207–15.

BROWN, S. F. (1938) Stuttering with relation to word accent and word position. *J. Abn. Soc. Psychol.* **33**, 112–20.

BROWN, S. F. (1945) The loci of stutterings in the speech sequence. *J. Sp. Dis.* **10**, 181–92.

BROWN, S. and MOREN, A. (1942) The frequency of stuttering in relation to word length during oral reading. *J. Sp. Dis.* **7**, 153–9.

BRUTTEN, E. J. (1957) A colorimetric anxiety measure of stuttering and expectancy adaptation. Ph.D. diss., Univ. Illinois.

BRUTTEN, E. J. (1963) Palmar sweat investigation of disfluency and expectancy adaptation. *J. Sp. Hear. Res.* **6**, 40–48.

BRUTTEN, E. J. and GRAY, B. B. (1961) Effect of word cue removal on adaptation and adjacency: a clinical paradigm. *J. Sp. Hear. Dis.* **26**, 385–9.

BRYNGELSON, B. (1935) Sidedness as an etiological factor in stuttering. *Pedagag. Semin.* **47**, 204–17.

BRYNGELSON, B. (1940) A study of laterality of stutterers and normal speakers. *J. Soc. Psychol.* **11**, 151–5.

BRYNGELSON, B., CHAPMAN, M. E. and HANSEN, O. K. (1950) *Know Yourself: A Workbook for those who Stutter*, Burgess Publishing Co., Minneapolis.

BRYNGELSON, B. and RUTHERFORD, B. (1937) A comparative study of laterality of stutterers and nonstutterers. *J. Sp. Dis.* **2**, 15–16.

CABANAS, R. (1954) Some findings in speech and voice therapy among mentally deficient children. *Folia Phoniat.* **6**, 34–37.

CARD, R. E. (1939) A study of allergy in relation to stuttering. *J. Sp. Dis.* **4**, 223–30.

CHERRY, C. and SAYERS, B. McA. (1956) Experiments upon the total inhibition of stammering by external control, and some clinical results. *J. Psychosomat. Res.* **1**, 233–46.

CHRISTENSEN, A. H. (1952) A quantitative study of personality dynamics in stuttering and nonstuttering siblings. *Sp. Monogr.* **19**, 187–8.

COHEN, E. (1952) A comparison of oral reading and spontaneous speech of stutterers with special reference to the adaptation and consistency effects. Ph.D. thesis, State Univ., Iowa.

CONNETT, MARIBEL (1955) Experimentally induced changes in the relative frequency of stuttering on a specified speech sound. In *Stuttering in Children and Adults*, ed. Wendell Johnson, Minnesota Press.

CONWAY, J. K. and QUARRINGTON, B. J. (1963) Positional effects in the stuttering of of contextually organized verbal material. *J. Abn. Soc. Psychol.* **67**, 299–303.

CORIAT, I. H. (1943) The psychoanalytic conception of stammering. *Nerv. Child.* **2**, 167–71.

CROSS, H. M. (1936) The motor capacities of stutterers. *Arch. Sp.* **1**, 112–32.

CULLINAN, W. I. (1963) Stability of adaptation in the oral performance of stutterers. *J. Sp. Hear. Res.* **6**, 70–83.

CULLINAN, W. L., PRATHER, E. M. and WILLIAMS, D. E. (1963) Comparison of procedures for scaling severity of stuttering. *J. Sp. Hear. Res.* **6**, 187–94.

CURTIS, J. (1942) A study of the effect of muscular exercise upon stuttering. *Sp. Monogr.* **9**, 61–74.

DAHLSTROM, W. G. and CRAVEN, D. D. (1952) The Minnesota Multiphasic Personality Inventory and stuttering phenomena in young adults. *Am. Psychol.* **7**, 341 (abstract).

DAHLSTROM, W. G. and WELSH, G. S. (1960) *An MMPI Handbook*, Minneapolis, Univ. Minn. Press.

DARLEY, F. L. (1940) A normative study of oral reading rate. M.A. Thesis, Univ. Iowa.

DAVIS, D. M. (1939) The relation of repetitions in the speech of young children to certain measures of language maturity and situational factors. Part I. *J. Sp. Dis.* **4**, 303–18.

DAVIS, D. M. (1940a) The relation of repetitions in the speech of young children to certain measures of language maturity and situational factors. Part II. *J. Sp. Dis.* **5**, 235–41.

DAVIS, D. M. (1940b) The relation of repetitions in the speech of young children to certain measures of language maturity and situational factors. Part III. *J. Sp. Dis.* **5**, 242–6.

DI CARLO, L. M., KATZ, J. and BATKIN, S. (1959) An exploratory investigation of the effect of meprobamate on stuttering behaviour. *J. Nerv. Ment. Dis.* **128**, 558–61.

DIEFFENBACH, J. F. (1841) *Memoir on the Radical Cure of Stuttering by a Surgical Operation* (translated from the German by Joseph Travers), London.

DIXON, C. (1947) The amount and rate of adaptation of stuttering in different oral reading situations. M.A. thesis, State Univ. Iowa.

DIXON, C. (1955) Stuttering adaptation in relation to assumed level of anxiety. In *Stuttering in Children and Adults*, Ed., W. Johnson, Univ. Minnesota Press, Minneapolis.

DOLL, B. A. (1940) *The Oseretsky Tests of Motor Proficiency*, Educational Publishers, Minneapolis.

DONOHUE, I. R. (1955) Stuttering adaptation during three hours of continuous oral reading. In *Stuttering in Children and Adults*, ed. W. Johnson, Univ. Minnesota Press, Minneapolis.

DOUGLASS, L. C. (1943) The study of laterally recorded EEGs of adult stutterers. *J. Exp. Psychol.* **32**, 247–65.

DOUGLASS, E. and QUARRINGTON, B. (1952) The differentiation of interiorized and exteriorized secondary stuttering. *J. Sp. Hear. Dis.* **17**, 377–85.

DOUST, J. W. L. (1956) Stress and psychopathology in stutterers. *Can. J. Psychol.* **10**, 31–37.

DOWNTON, W. (1955) The effect of instructions concerning mode of stuttering on the breathing of stutterers. In *Stuttering in Children and Adults*, ed. W. Johnson, Univ. Minnesota Press, Minneapolis.

EISENSON, J. (1937) A note on the perseverating tendency in stutterers. *Pedagog. Semin.* **50**, 195–8.

EISENSON, J. (1958) A perseveration theory of stuttering. In *Stuttering: A Symposium*, ed., J. Eisenson, Harper & Bros., New York.

EISENSON, J. and HOROWITZ, ESTHER (1945) The influence of propositionality on stuttering. *J. Sp. Dis.* **10**, 193–7.

EISENSON, J. and WELLS, C. (1942) A study of the influence communication responsibility in a choral speech situation for stutterers. *J. Sp. Dis.* **7**, 259–62.

ENGLISH, H. B. and ENGLISH, AVA (1958) *A Comprehensive Dictionary of Psychological and Psychoanalytical Terms*, Longmans, New York.

FALCK, F. J. (1955) Interrelationships among certain behavioural characteristics, age, sex and duration of therapy in a group of stutterers. Ph.D. diss., Penn State Univ.

FENICHEL, O. (1945) *The Psychoanalytic Theory of Neurosis*, Norton, New York.

FIEDLER, F. E. and WEPMAN, J. (1951) An exploratory investigation of the self-concept of stutterers. *J. Sp. Dis.* **16**, 110–14.

FIERMAN, ELLA (1955) The role of cues in stuttering adaptation. In *Stuttering in Children and Adults*, ed., W. Johnson, Univ. Minnesota Press, Minneapolis.

FINKELSTEIN, P. and WEISBERGER, S. (1954) The motor proficiency of stutterers. *J. Sp. Hear. Dis.* **19**, 52–58.

FISHMAN, H. H. (1937) A study of the efficacy of negative practice as a corrective for stammering. *J. Sp. Dis.* **2**, 67–72.

FLANAGAN, J. C. (1935) *Factor Analysis in the Study of Personality*, Stanford Univ. Calif., Stanford Univ. Press.

FLANAGAN, B., GOLDIAMOND, I. and AZRIN, N. H. (1958) Operant stuttering: the control of stuttering behaviour through response-contingent consequences. *J. Exp. Anal. Behav.* **1**, 173–8.

FLETCHER, J. M. (1928) *The Problem of Stuttering*, Longmans, New York.

Font, M. M. (1955) A comparison of the free associations of stutterers and nonstutterers. In *Stuttering in Children and Adults*, ed., W. Johnson. Univ. Minnesota Press, Minneapolis.

Fossler, H. (1930) Disturbances in breathing during stuttering. *Psychol. Monogr.* **40**, 1–32.

Fransella, Fay (1965a) The effects of imposed rhythm and certain aspects of personality on the speech of stutterers. Ph.D. thesis, Univ. London.

Fransella, Fay (1965b) An experimental evaluation of the speech correction semantic differential. *Sp. Monogr.* **32**, 448–51.

Fransella, Fay (1967) Rhythm as a distractor in the modification of stuttering. *Behav. Res. Ther.* **5**, 253–5.

Fransella, Fay (1968) Self concepts and the stutterer. *J. Psychiat.* (in press).

Fransella, Fay and Beech, H. R. (1965) An experimental analysis of the effect of rhythm on the speech of stutterers. *Behav. Res. Ther.* **3**, 195–201.

Fraser, M. (1963) *Stuttering Words* (revised), Speech Foundation of America, 152 Lombardy Road, Memphis, Tennessee.

Freund, H. (1934) Ueber Inneres Stottern. *Z. ges. Neurol. Psychiat.* **151**, 585–98.

Frick, J. V. (1955) Spontaneous recovery of the stuttering response as a function of the degree of adaptation. In *Stuttering in Children and Adults*, ed., W. Johnson, Univ. Minnesota Press, Minneapolis.

Froeschels, E. (1941) Differences in the symptomatology of stuttering in the U.S. and in Europe. *J. Sp. Dis.* **6**, 45–46.

Froeschels, E. (1950) A technique for stutterers—"ventriloquism", *J. Sp. Hear. Dis.* **15**, 336–7.

Gardner, W. H. (1937) The study of the pupillary reflex, with special reference to stuttering. *Psychol. Monogr.* **49**, 1–31.

Giolas, T. G. and Williams, D. E. (1958) Children's reactions to nonfluencies in adult speech. *J. Sp. Hear. Res.* **1**, 86–93.

Glaser, E. M. (1936) Possible relationship between stuttering and endocrine malfunctioning. *J. Sp. Dis.* **1**, 81–89.

Glasner, P. (1949) Personality characteristics and emotional problems in stutterers under the age of five. *J. Sp. Hear. Dis.* **14**, 135–8.

Glasner, P. and Vermilyea, F. D. (1953) An investigation of the definition and use of the diagnosis, "primary stuttering". *J. Sp. Hear. Dis.* **18**, 161–7.

Glauber, J. P. (1958) The psychoanalysis of stuttering. In *Stuttering: A Symposium*, ed., Eisenson, J. Harper Bros., New York.

Goldfarb, W. and Braunstein, P. (1958) Reactions to delayed auditory feedback in schizophrenic children. In *Psychopathology of Communication*, eds., P. H. Hoch and J. Zubin, Grune & Stratton, New York.

Goldiamond, I. (1965) Stuttering and fluency as manipulable operant response classes. In *Research in Behaviour Modifications*, eds. L. Krasner and L. P. Ullman, Holt, Rinehart & Winston, New York.

Goldman-Eisler, F. (1958) Speech production and the probability of words in context. *Quart. J. Exp. Psychol.* **10**, 96–106.

Goldman, R. and Shames, G. H. (1964a) A study of goal-setting behaviour of parents of stutterers and parents of nonstutterers. *J. Sp. Hear. Dis.* **29**, 192–4.

Goldman, R. and Shames, G. H. (1964b) Comparisons of the goals that parents of stutterers and parents of nonstutterers set for their children. *J. Sp. Hear. Dis.* **29**, 381–9.

Golub, A. (1955) The cumulative effect of constant and varying reading material on stuttering adaptation, In *Stuttering in Children and Adults*, ed. W. Johnson, Univ. Minnesota Press, Minneapolis.

GOODSTEIN, L. D. (1958) Functional speech disorders and personality: a survey of the research. *J. Sp. Hear. Res.* **1**, 359–76.

GOODSTEIN, L. D., MARTIRE, J. G. and SPIELBERGER, C. D. (1955) The relationship between "achievement imagery" and stuttering behaviour in college males. *Proc. Iowa Acad. Sci.* **62**, 399–404.

GORDON, M. B. (1928) Stammering produced by thyroid medication. *Am. J. Med. Sci.* **175**, 360.

GOSS, A. E. (1952) Stuttering behaviour and anxiety as a function of the duration of stimulus words. *J. Abn. Soc. Psychol.* **47**, 38–50.

GOSS, A. E. (1956) Stuttering behaviour and anxiety as a function of experimental training. *J. Sp. Hear. Dis.* **21**, 343–51.

GRAF, ODNY (1955) Incidence of stuttering among twins. In *Stuttering in Children and Adults*, ed. W. Johnson, Univ. Minnesota Press, Minneapolis.

GRAY, B. B. (1961) A palmar sweat investigation of response adaptation. M.A. thesis, Southern Illinois Univ.

GRAY, B. B. (1965a) Theoretical approximations of stuttering adaptation. *Behav. Res. Ther.* **3**, 171–85.

GRAY, B. B. (1965b) Theoretical approximations of stuttering adaptation: statement of predictive accuracy. *Behav. Res. Ther.* **3**, 221–7.

GRAY, B. B. (1966) Personal communication.

GRAY, B. B. and BRUTTEN, E. J. (1965) The relationship between anxiety, fatigue and spontaneous recovery in stuttering. *Behav. Res. Ther.* **2**, 251–9.

GRAY, B. B. and KARMEN, JANE (1966) The relationship between nonverbal anxiety and stuttering adaptation. *J. Sp. Hear. Res.* In Press.

GREENSPOON, J. (1962) Verbal conditioning and clinical psychology. In *Experimental Foundations of Clinical Psychology*, Ed. A. J. Bachrach, Basic Books, New York.

GREGORY, H. H. (1964) Stuttering and auditory central nervous system disorder. *J. Sp. Hear. Res.* **7**, 335–41.

GUTZMANN, H. (1912) *Sprachheilkunde*, Berlin.

HACKETT, J. D., HOFFMAN, M., MACLEOD, A. W. and SURTEES, R. (1958) A study of the effects of chlorpromazine as an aid to therapy for stuttering with a one-year follow-up. *Proc. ASHA Convention*, New York.

HAGEMANN, HENRIETTE (1845) *Die untruegliche Heilung des Stotter- und Stammel-Ubbels*, Breslau.

HAHN, E. F. (1942) A study of the relationship between stuttering occurrence of two phonetic factors in oral reading. *J. Sp. Dis.* **7**, 143–51.

HALE, L. L. (1951) A consideration of thiamin supplement in prevention of stuttering in preschool children. *J. Sp. Hear. Dis.* **16**, 327–33.

HALLE (1900) Ueber Storungen der Athmung bei Stottern. *Monatschr. f. Sprachheilkunde* **10**, 225.

HANEY, R. H. (1950) Motives implied by the act of stuttering as revealed by prolonged experimental projection. Doct. diss., Univ. Southern Calif.

HARMS, M. A. and MALONE, J. Y. (1939) The relationship of hearing acuity to stammering. *J. Sp. Dis.* **4**, 363.

HARRIS, W. E. (1940) A study of the adaptation effect in stuttering. M.A. thesis, State Univ. Iowa.

HARRIS, W. E. (1942) Studies in the psychology of stuttering. XVII. A study of the transfer of the adaptation effect in stuttering. *J. Sp. Dis.* **7**, 209–221

HAUSDORFER, O. (1898) *Warum stottere ich?*, Breslau.

HEJNA, R. F. (1955) A study of the loci of stuttering in spontaneous speech. Ph.D. diss., Northwestern Univ.

HELTMAN, H. J. (1940) Contradictory evidence in handedness and stuttering. *J. Sp. Dis.* **5**, 327–31.

HERBERT, M. (1966) Personal communication.
HILL, H. (1944) Stuttering. I. A critical review and evaluation of bio-chemical investigations. *J. Sp. Dis.* **9**, 245–61.
HILL, H. (1954) An experimental study of disorganization of speech and manual responses in normal subjects. *J. Sp. Hear. Dis.* **1**, 295–305.
HOGEWIND, F. (1940) Medical treatment of stuttering. *J. Sp. Dis.* **5**, 203–8.
HOLLIDAY, AUDREY (1959) Effect of meprobamate on stuttering. *Northwest Med.* **58**, 837–41.
HOLLINGSWORTH, H. L. (1939) Chewing as a technique of relaxation. *Science* **90**, 385–7.
HOLLISTER, L. E. (1955) Advantages of placebos and the double-blind method for evaluating drugs used in psychiatry. *Proc. Acad. Psychosomat. Med.*, New York City.
HONIG, P. (1947) The stutterer acts it out. *J. Sp. Dis.* **12**, 105–9.
HULL, C. L. (1943) *Principles of Behaviour*, Appleton–Century–Crofts, New York.
HUNSLEY, Y. L. (1937) Dysintegration in the speech musculature of stutterers during the production of a nonverbal temporal pattern. *Psychol. Monogr.* **49**, 32–49.
INGERBREGSTEN, E. (1936) Some experimental contributions to the psychology and psychopathology of stuttering. *Am. J. Orthopsychiat.* **6**, 630–51.
ITARD, (1817) Mémoire sur le bégaiement. *J. Universel des sciences medicales*, **VIII**.
JAMISON, DOROTHY (1955) Spontaneous recovery of the stuttering response as a function of the time following adaptation. In *Stuttering in Children and Adults*, Ed. W. Johnson, Univ. Minnesota Press, Minneapolis.
JASPER, H. H. (1932) A laboratory study of diagnostic indices of bilateral neuro-muscular organization in stutterers and normal speakers. *Psychol. Monogr.* **43**, 72–174.
JASPER, H. H. and MURRAY, E. (1932) A study of the eye-movements of stutterers during oral reading. *J. Exp. Psychol.* **15**, 528–38.
JOHNSON, W. (1932) *The Influence of Stuttering on the Personality*, Univ. Iowa Press, Studies in Child Welfare, Vol. 5, No. 5, Iowa City.
JOHNSON, W. (1942) A study of the onset and development of stuttering. *J. Sp. Dis.* **7**, 251–7.
JOHNSON, W. (1946) *People in Quandries: the Semantics of Personal Adjustment*, Harpers, New York.
JOHNSON, W. (Ed.) (1955) The time, the place and the problem. In *Stuttering in Children and Adults*, Univ. Minnesota Press, Minneapolis.
JOHNSON, W. (Ed.) (1955) *Stuttering in Children and Adults*, Univ. Minnesota Press, Minneapolis.
JOHNSON, W. and AINSWORTH, S. (1938) Studies in the psychology of stuttering. X. Constancy of loci of expectancy of stuttering. *J. Sp. Dis.* **3**, 101–4.
JOHNSON, W. and BROWN, S. (1935) Stuttering in relation to various speech sounds. *Qrt. J. Sp.* **21**, 481–96.
JOHNSON, W., BROWN, S. F., CURTIS, J. F., EDNEY, C. W. and KEASTER, J. (1956) *Speech Handicapped School Children*, 2nd ed., Harper and Row, New York.
JOHNSON, W., DARLEY, F. L. and SPRIESTERSBACH, D. C. (1963) *Diagnostic Methods in Speech Pathology*, Harper & Row, New York.
JOHNSON, W. and associates (1959) *The Onset of Stuttering*, Minnesota Press, Minneapolis.
JOHNSON, W. and INNESS, M. (1939) Studies in the psychology of stuttering. XIII. A statistical analysis of the adaptation and consistency effects in relation to stuttering. *J. Sp. Dis.* **4**, 76–86.

JOHNSON, W. and KNOTT, J. (1937) Studies in the psychology of stuttering. I. The distribution of moments of stuttering in successive readings of the same material. *J. Sp. Dis.* **2**, 17–19.

JOHNSON, W. and ROSEN, L. (1937) Studies in the psychology of stuttering. VII. Effect of certain changes in speech pattern upon frequency of stuttering. *J. Sp. Dis.* **2**, 105–9.

JOHNSON, W. and SINN, A. (1937) Studies in the psychology of stuttering. V. Frequency of stuttering with expectation of stuttering controlled. *J. Sp. Dis.* **2**, 98–100.

JOHNSON, W. and SOLOMON, A. (1937) Studies in the psychology of stuttering. IV. A quantitative study of expectation of stuttering as a process involving a low degree of consciousness. *J. Sp. Dis.* **2**, 95–97.

JOHNSON, W., STEARNS, G. and WARWEG, E. (1933) Chemical factors and the stuttering spasm, *Quart. J. Sp.* **19**, 409–14.

JOHNSON, W., YOUNG, M. A., SAHS, A. L. and BEDELL, G. N. (1959) Effects of hyperventilation and tetany on the speech fluency of stutterers and non-stutterers. *J. Sp. Hear. Res.* **2**, 203–15.

JONES, E. L. (1955) Explorations of experimental extinction and spontaneous recovery in stuttering. In *Stuttering in Children and Adults*, ed. W. Johnson, Univ. Minnesota Press, Minneapolis.

JONES, R. K. (1966) Observations on stammering after localized cerebral injury. *J. Neurol. Neurosurg. Psychiat.* **29**, 192–5.

KAPOS, E. and FATTU, N. (1957) Behavioural rigidity in speech-handicapped children. *J. Sp. Hear. Dis.* **22**, 707–13.

KAPOS, E. and STANDLEE, L. S. (1958) Behavioural rigidity in adult stutterers. *J. Sp. Hear. Res.* **1**, 294–6.

KARLIN, I. W. and SOBEL, A. E. (1940) A comparative study of the blood chemistry of stutterers and nonstutterers. *Sp. Monogr.* **7**, 75–84.

KARMEN, JANE L. (1964) A comparison between generalized anxiety adjustment and adaptation of stuttering behaviour. Ph.D. diss., Univ. Arizona.

KASTEIN, S. (1947) The chewing method of treating stuttering. *J. Sp. Dis.* **12**, 195–8.

KELLY, G. A. (1932) Some common factors in reading and speech disabilities. *Psychol. Monogr.* **43**, 175–203.

KELLY, G. A. (1955) *The Psychology of Personal Constructs*, Vols. 1 and 2, Norton, New York.

KENNEDY, A. M. and WILLIAMS, D. A. (1938) Association of stammering and the allergic diathesis. *Brit. Med. J.* **2**, 1306–9.

KENT, LOUISE (1961) Carbon dioxide therapy as a medical treatment of stuttering. *J. Sp. Hear. Dis.* **26**, 268–71.

KENT, LOUISE (1963) The use of tranquilizers in the treatment of stuttering. *J. Sp. Hear. Dis.* **28**, 288–94.

KENT, LOUISE and WILLIAMS, D. E. (1959) Use of meprobamate as an adjunct to stuttering therapy. *J. Sp. Hear. Dis.* **24**, 64–69.

KERN, A. (1932) Der Einflus des Hörens auf das Stottern. *Arch. Psychiat.* **97**, 429–49.

KIMMELL, M. (1938) Studies in the psychology of stuttering. IX. The nature and effects of stutterers' avoidance reaction. *J. Sp. Dis.* **3**, 95–100.

KING, P. T. (1953) Perseverating factors in a stuttering and nonstuttering population. Ph.D. diss., Penn. State Univ.

KLOPFER, B., KIRKNER, F. J., WISHAM, W., BAKER, G., MINDESS, H., SHEEHAN, J. G., SPIEGELMAN, M. and SEACAT, G. (1951) Symposium on the rating of unused ego-strength by the Rorschach Method. *J. Proj. Tech.* **15**, 421–4.

KNOTT, J. R., CORRELL, R. E. and SHEPHERD, J. N. (1959) Frequency analysis of electroencephalograms of stutterers and nonstutterers. *J. Sp. Hear. Res.* **2**, 74–80.

KNOTT, J. R., JOHNSON, W. and WEBSTER, M. J. (1937) Studies in the psychology of stuttering. II. A quantitative evaluation of expectation of stuttering in relation to the occurrence of stuttering. *J. Sp. Dis.* **2**, 20–22.

KNOTT, J. R. and TJOSSEM, T. D. (1943) Bilateral electroencephalograms from normal speakers and stutterers. *J. Exp. Psychol.* **35**, 356–62.

KOPP, G. A. (1934) Metabolic studies of stutterers. I. Biochemical study of blood composition. *Sp. Monogr.* **1**, 117–30.

KOPP, HELENE (1943) The relationship of stuttering to motor disturbances. *Nerv. Child* **2**, 107–16.

KRASNER, L. (1958) Studies on the conditioning of verbal behaviour. *Psychol. Bull.* **55**, 148–70.

KRUGMAN, M. (1946) Psychosomatic study of fifty stuttering children. Round Table IV, Rorschach Study. *Am. J. Orthopsychiat.* **16**, 127–33.

LANYON, R. I. (1965) The relationship of adaptation and consistency to improvement in stuttering therapy. *J. Sp. Hear. Res.* **8**, 263–9.

LANYON, R. I. (1966) The MMPI and prognosis in stuttering therapy. *J. Sp. Hear. Dis.* **31**, 186–91.

LEE, B. S. (1950) Effects of delayed speech feedback. *J. Acoust. Soc. Am.* **22**, 824–6.

LEE, B. S. (1951) Artificial stutter. *J. Sp. Hear. Dis.* **16**, 53–55.

LEMERT, E. M. (1953) Some Indians who stutter. *J. Sp. Hear. Dis.* **18**, 168–74.

LEMERT, E. M. and VAN RIPER, C. (1944) The use of psychodrama in the treatment of speech defects. *Sociometry* **7**, 190–5.

LEUTENEGGER, R. (1957) Adaptation and recovery in the oral readings of stutterers. *J. Sp. Hear. Dis.* **22**, 276–87.

LIEBMAN, M. (1956) The test–retest reliability of adaptation and consistency scores. M.A. Thesis, Brooklyn College.

LIGHTFOOT, C. (1948) Serial identification of colors by stutterers. *J. Sp. Hear. Dis.* **16**, 114–19.

LILLEHEI, J. P. and BALKE, B. (1955) *Studies of Hyperventilation*, U.S.A.F. School of Aviation Medicine, Randolph Field, Texas.

LINDSLEY, D. B. (1940) Bilateral differences in brain potentials from the two cerebral hemispheres in relation to laterality and stuttering. *J. Exp. Psychol.* **26**, 211–25.

LOUTIT, C. M. and HALLS, E. C. (1936) Survey of speech defects. *J. Sp. Hear. Dis.* **1**, 73.

LOVE, W. R. (1955) The effect of pentobarbital (nembutal) and amphetamine sulphate (benzedrine) on the severity of stuttering. In *Stuttering in Children and Adults*, Ed. W. Johnson. Univ. Minnesota Press, Minneapolis.

LOWINGER, L. (1952) The psychodynamics of stuttering: an evaluation of the factors of aggression and guilt feelings in a group of institutionalized children. Ph.D. diss., New York Univ.

LUCHSINGER, H. (1940) Die Sprache und Stimme von ein-und Zweieigen Zwillingen in Beziehung zur Motorik und zum Erbcharacter. *Julius Kraus, Stiftung fur Vererbungsforschung, Soziatanthropologie und Rassen-hygiene, Archiv., Zurich*, **15**, 15.

LUPER, H. L. (1954) The consistency of selected aspects of behaviour in the repetitions of stuttered words. Ph.D. diss., Ohio State Univ.

LUPER, H. L. (1959) Relative severity of stuttering ratings from visual and auditory presentations of the same speech sample. *Southern Sp. J.* **25**, 107–14.

MADDOX, J. (1938) Studies in the psychology of stuttering. VIII. The role of visual cues in the precipitation of moments of stuttering. *J. Sp. Dis.* **3**, 90–94.

MADISON, L. R. and NORMAN, R. D. (1952) A comparison of the performance of stutterers and nonstutterers on the Rosenzweig picture-frustration test. *J. Clin. Psychol.* **8,** 179–83.

MARAIST, J. A. and HUTTON, C. (1957) Effects of auditory masking upon the speech of stutterers. *J. Sp. Hear. Dis.* **22,** 385–9.

MARKS, P. A. and SEEMAN, W. (1963) *Actuarial Description of Abnormal Personality,* Williams & Wilkins, Baltimore.

MARTIN, R. (1962) Stuttering and preservation in children, *J. Sp. Hear. Res.* **5,** 332–9.

MAST, V. R. (1951) Level of aspiration as a method of studying the personality of adult stutterers. M.A. diss., Univ. Michigan.

McCROSKY, R. (1957) Effect of speech on metabolism: a comparison between stutterers and nonstutterers. *J. Sp. Hear. Dis.* **22,** 46–52.

McDOWELL, E. (1928) *Educational and Emotional Adjustments of Stuttering Children,* Columbia Univ., Teachers College Contributors to Education, No. 314.

MEDUNA, L. J. (1950) *Carbon Dioxide Therapy,* 1st ed., Charles C. Thomas, Springfield, Illinois.

MEFFERT, M. L. (1956) The effect of serpasil (reserpine) on the severity of stuttering. M.A. thesis, Univ. Virginia.

MEIKLE, LOUISE (1962) An investigation of spontaneous recovery under two conditions of drive. M.A. thesis, Southern Illinois Univ.

MELTZER, H. (1944) Personality differences between stuttering and nonstuttering children as indicated by the Rorschach test. *J. Psychol.* **17,** 39–59.

MÉTRAUX, R. W. (1950) Speech profiles of the pre-school child 18 to 54 months. *J. Sp. Hear. Dis.* **15,** 37–53.

MEYER, V. and MAIR, J. M. M. (1963) A new technique to control stammering: a preliminary report. *Behav. Res. Ther.* **1,** 251–4.

MILISEN, R. (1938) Frequency of stuttering with anticipation of stuttering controlled. *J. Sp. Dis.* **3,** 207–14.

MILISEN, R. (1957) Methods of evaluation and diagnosis of speech disorders. Chap. 8 in Travis, L. E. *Handbook of Speech Pathology,* Appleton–Century–Crofts Inc., New York.

MILLER, F. J. W., COURT, S. D. M., WALTON, W. S. and KNOX, E. G. (1960) *Growing up in Newcastle-upon-Tyne,* Oxford Univ. Press, London.

MILLER, G. A. (1951) *Language and Communication,* McGraw-Hill, New York.

MILLER, G. R. and HEWGILL, M. A. (1964) The effect of variations in nonfluency on audience ratings of source credibility. *Qrt. J. Sp.* **50,** 36–44.

MILLS, A. W. and STREIT, H. (1942) Report of a speech survey, Holyoke, Massachusetts. *J. Sp. Dis.* **7,** 161.

MITCHELL, B. A. (1955) An analysis of the effect of reserpine on adult stutterers. M.A. diss., Western Michigan Univ.

MONCUR, J. P. (1952) Parental domination in stuttering. *J. Sp. Hear. Dis.* **17,** 155–65.

MOORE, W. E. (1946) Hypnosis in a system of therapy of stutterers. *J. Sp. Dis.* **11,** 117–22.

MORAVEK, M. and LANGOVA, A. (1962) Some electrophysiological findings among stutterers and clutterers. *Folia Phoniat.* **14,** 395–416.

MORGENSTERN, J. (1956) Socio-economic factors in stuttering. *J. Sp. Hear. Dis.* **21,** 25–33.

MORLEY, D. E. (1952) A ten-year survey of speech disorders among university students. *J. Sp. Dis.* **17,** 25.

MORLEY, D. E. (1957) *The Development and Disorders of Speech in Childhood,* Livingstone, Edinburgh.

MOSER, H. M. (1938) A qualitative analysis of eye movements during stuttering. *J. Sp. Dis.* **3**, 131–9.

MOWRER, O. H. (1938) Preparatory set (expectancy)—a determinant in motivation and conditioning. *Psychol. Rev.* **45**, 62–81.

MOWRER, O. H. (1940) Preparatory set (expectancy)—some methods of measurement. *Psychol. Monogr.* **52**, whole no. 233.

MURPHY, A. T. and FITZSIMONS, RUTH (1960) *Stuttering and Personality Dynamics*, Roland, New York.

MURRAY, E. (1932) Dysintegration of breathing and eye movements in stuttering during silent reading and reasoning. *Psychol. Monogr.* **43**, 218–75.

NEELEY, J. N. (1961) A study of the speech behaviour of stutterers and non-stutterers under normal and delayed auditory feedback. *J. Sp. Hear. Dis.*, Monogr. Suppl. No. 7.

NELSON, S. F., HUNTER, N. and WALTER, M. (1945) Stuttering in twin types. *J. Sp. Dis.* **10**, 335–43.

NEWMAN, H. H., FREEMAN, F. N. and HOLZINGER, K. J. (1937) *Twins: A study of Heredity and Environment*, Chicago.

NEWMAN, P. W. (1954) A study of adaptation and recovery of the stuttering response in self-formulated speech. *J. Sp. Hear. Dis.* **19**, 450–8.

NEWMAN, P. W. (1963) Adaptation performances of individual stutterers: implications for research. *J. Sp. Hear. Res.* **6**, 292–4.

NICOL, M. A. and MILLER, R. M. (1959) Word redundancy in written English. *Austral. J. Psychol.* **11**, 81–91.

ORTON, S. T. (1928) A physiological theory of reading disability and stuttering in children. *New Eng. J. Med.* **199.**

OSERETSKY, N. (1931) *Psychomotorik. Methoden zur Untersuchung der Motorik*, Leipzig.

OSGOOD, C. E., SUCI, G. J., TANNENBAUM, P. H. (1957) *The Measurement of Meaning*, Urbana, Ill., Univ of Illinois Press.

OWEN, T. and STEMMERMANN, P. (1947) Electric convulsive therapy in stammering. *J. Psychiat.* **104**, 410–13.

OXTOBY, E. T. (1955) Frequency of stuttering in relation to induced modifications following expectancy of stuttering. In *Stuttering in Children and Adults*, ed. W. Johnson, Univ. Minnesota Press, Minneapolis.

PALASEK, J. R. and CURTIS, W. S. (1960) Sugar placebos and stuttering. *J. Sp. Hear. Res.* **3**, 223–6.

PALMER, M. and GILLETT, A. M. (1938) Sex differences in the cardiac rhythms of stutterers. *J. Sp. Dis.* **3**, 3–12.

PALMER, M. and OSBORN, C. D. (1940) A study of tongue pressures of speech defective and normal speaking individuals. *J. Sp. Dis.* **5**, 133–40.

PATTIE, F. A. and KNIGHT, B. B. (1944) Why does the speech of stutterers improve in chorus reading? *J. Abn. Soc. Psychol.* **39**, 362–7.

PEACHER, W. G. and HARRIS, W. E. (1946) Speech disorders in World War II. VIII. Stuttering. *J. Sp. Dis.* **11**, 303.

PEINS, MARYANN (1961) Adaptation effect and spontaneous recovery in stuttering expectancy. *J. Sp. Hear. Res.* **4**, 91–99.

PENFIELD, W. and ROBERTS, L. (1959) *Speech and Brain Mechanisms*, Princeton Univ. Press, Princeton, New Jersey.

PITRELLI, F. R. (1948) Psychosomatic and Rorschach aspects of stuttering. *Psychiat. Quart.* **22**, 175–94.

PIZZAT, F. J. (1949) A personality study of college stutterers. M.S. diss., Univ. Pittsburg.

PORTER, H. V. K. (1939) Studies in the psychology of stuttering. XIV. Stuttering phenomena in relation to size and personnel of audience. *J. Sp. Dis.* **4**, 323–33.

PRATHER, E. M. (1960) Scaling defectiveness of articulation by direct magnitude-estimation. *J. Sp. Hear. Res.* **3**, 380–92.

QUARRINGTON, B. (1953) The performance of stutterers on the Rosenzweig picture-frustration test. *J. Clin. Psychol.* **2**, 189–92.

QUARRINGTON, B. (1959) Measures of stuttering adaptation. *J. Sp. Hear. Res.* **2**, 105–12.

QUARRINGTON, B. (1965) Stuttering as a function of the information value and sentence position of words. *J. Abn. Psychol.* **70**, 221–4.

QUARRINGTON, B., CONWAY, J. K. and SIEGEL, N. (1962) An experimental study of some properties of stuttered words. *J. Sp. Hear. Res.* **5**, 388–94.

QUARRINGTON, B. and DOUGLASS, E. (1960) Audibility avoidance in nonvocalized stutterers. *J. Sp. Hear. Dis.* **25**, 358–65.

RAHN, H. and associates (1946) The effects of hypocapnia on performance. *J. Aviat. Med.* **17**, 164.

RAIMY, V. C. (1948) Self-reference in counselling interviews. *J. Consult. Psychol.* **12**, 153–63.

RANEY, E. T. (1935) A phi-test for the determination of lateral dominance involving the visual perception of movement. *Psychol. Bull.* **32**, 740.

RANEY, E. T. (1938) Brain potentials and lateral dominance in identical twins. *J. Exp. Psychol.* **24**, 21.

RAZDOLSKY, V. A. (1965) On the speech of stutterers when alone. *Zhurnal Nevropatologii i Psikhiatrii*, **65**, 1717–20.

REID, L. D. (1946) Some facts about stuttering. *J. Sp. Dis.* **11**, 3.

RHEINBERGER, M. B., KARLIN, I. W. and BERMAN, A. B. (1943) Electroencephalographic and laterality studies of stuttering and nonstuttering children. *Nerv. Child.* **2**, 117–33.

RICHARDSON, L. H. (1944) A personality study of stutterers and nonstutterers. *J. Sp. Dis.* **9**, 152–60.

RITZMAN, C. H. (1942) A comparative cardiovascular and metabolic study of stutterers and nonstutterers. *J. Sp. Dis.* **7**, 367–73.

RITZMAN, C. H. (1943) A cardiovascular and metabolic study of stutterers and nonstutterers. *J. Sp. Dis.* **8**, 161–82.

ROBBINS, S. (1935) The role of rhythm in the correction of stammering. *Qrt. J. Sp.* **21**, 331–43.

ROGERS, C. R. (1951) *Client-centered Therapy*, Houghton Mifflin, Boston.

ROSENBERG, S. and CURTIS, J. (1954) The effect of stuttering on the behaviour of the listener. *J. Abn. Soc. Psychol.* **49**, 355–61.

ROSS, F. L. (1955) A comparative study of stutterers and nonstutterers on a psychomotor discrimination task. In *Stuttering in Children and Adults*, ed. W. Johnson, Univ. Minnesota Press, Minneapolis.

ROTTER, J. B. (1942) Level of aspiration as a method of studying personality. II. Development and evaluation of a controlled method. *J. Exp. Psychol.* **31**, 410–22.

ROTTER, J. B. (1947) Level of aspiration as a method of studying personality. *Psychol. Rev.* **49**, 463–74.

ROTTER, J. B. (1955) A study of the motor integration of stutterers and non-stutterers. In *Stuttering in Children and Adults*, ed. W. Johnson. Univ. Minnesota Press, Minneapolis.

ROUSEY, C. L. (1958) Stuttering severity during prolonged spontaneous speech. *J. Sp. Hear. Res.* **1**, 40–47.

ROUSEY, C. L., GEOTZINGER, C. P. and DIRKS, D. (1959) Sound localization ability of normal, stuttering, neurotic and hemiplegic subjects. *A.M.A. Arch. Gen. Psychiat.* **1**, 640–5.

SANDER, E. K. (1961) Reliability of the Iowa speech disfluency test. *J. Sp. Hear. Dis.*, Monogr. Suppl., **7**, 21–30.

SANDER, E. K. (1963) Frequency of syllable repetitions and "stutterer" judgements. *J. Sp. Hear. Dis.* **28**, 19–30.

SANDER, E. K. (1965) Comments on investigating listener reaction to speech disfluency, *J. Sp. Hear. Dis.* **30**, 159–65.

SANTOSTEFANO, S. (1960) Anxiety and hostility. *J. Sp. Hear. Res.* **3**, 337–47.

SCHLANGER, B. B. and GOTTSLEBEN, R. H. (1957) Analysis of speech defects among the institutionalized mentally retarded. *J. Sp. Hear. Dis.* **22**, 98.

SCHLESINGER, I. M., FORTE, M., FRIED, B. and MELKMAN, RACHEL (1965) Stuttering, information load and response strength. *J. Sp. Hear. Dis.* **30**, 32–36.

SCHUELL, H. (1946) Sex differences in relation to stuttering. Part I. *J. Sp. Dis.* **11**, 277–98.

SCHUELL, H. (1947) Sex differences in relation to stuttering. Part II. *J. Sp. Dis.* **12**, 23–28.

SEEMAN, M. (1939) The significance of twin pathology for the investigation of speech disorders. *Arch. für die Gesamte Phonetik* **1**, 88.

SETH, G. (1934) An experimental study of the control of the mechanisms of speech, and in particular that of respiration, in stuttering subjects. *Brit. J. Psychol.* **24**, 375–88.

SHAMES, G. H. (1949) The relationship between the attitude toward stuttering of secondary stutterers and several of their personality characteristics. M.S. diss., Univ. Pittsburgh.

SHAMES, G. H. (1952) An investigation of prognosis and evaluation in speech therapy. *J. Sp. Hear. Dis.* **17**, 386–92.

SHAMES, G. H. (1953) A utilisation of adaptation phenomena in therapy for stuttering. *J. Sp. Hear. Dis.* **18**, 256–7.

SHAMES, G. H. and SHERRICK, C. E. (1963) A discussion of nonfluency and stuttering as operant behaviour. *J. Sp. Hear. Dis.* **28**, 3–18.

SHANE, M. L. (1955) Effect on stuttering of alteration in auditory feedback. In *Stuttering in Children and Adults*, ed. W. Johnson, Univ. Minnesota Press, Minneapolis.

SHEARER, W. M. (1961) A theoretical consideration of the self-concept and body-image in stuttering therapy. *Am. Sp. Hear. Assoc.* **3**, 115–16.

SHEARER, W. M. and SIMMONS, F. B. (1965) Middle ear activity during speech in normal speakers and stutterers. *J. Sp. Hear. Res.* **8**, 203–7.

SHEEHAN, J. G. (1951) The modification of stuttering through nonreinforcement. *J. Abn. Soc. Psychol.* **46**, 51–63.

SHEEHAN, J. G. (1954) An integration of psychotherapy and speech therapy through a conflict theory of stuttering. *J. Sp. Hear. Dis.* **19**, 474–82.

SHEEHAN, J. G. (1958a) Projective studies of stuttering. *J. Sp. Hear. Dis.* **23**, 18–25.

SHEEHAN, J. G. (1958b) Conflict theory of stuttering. In *Stuttering: A Symposium*, ed. J. Eisenson, Harper Bros., New York.

SHEEHAN, J. G., CORTESE, P. A., HADLEY, R. G. (1962). Guilt, shame, and tension, in graphic projections of stuttering. *J. Sp. Hear. Dis.* **27**, 129–39).

SHEEHAN, J. G., FREDERICK, C. J., ROSEVEAR, W. H. and SPIEGELMAN, M. (1954) A validity study of the Rorschach prognostic rating scale. *J. Proj. Tech.* **18**, 233–9.

SHEEHAN, J. G. and MARTYN, MARGARET M. (1966) Spontaneous recovery from stuttering. *J. Sp. Hear. Res.* **9**, 121–35.

SHEEHAN, J. G. and VOAS, R. B. (1954) Tension patterns during stuttering in relation to conflict, fear-reduction, and reinforcement. *Sp. Monogr.* 21, 272–9.

SHEEHAN, J. G. and ZELEN, S. L. (1951) A level of aspiration study of stutterers. *Am. Psychol.* 6, 500 (abstract).

SHEEHAN, J. G. and ZELEN, S. L. (1955) Level of aspiration in stutterers and nonstutterers. *J. Abn. Soc. Psychol.* 51, 83–86.

SHERMAN, D. (1952) Clinical and experimental use of the Iowa scale of severity of stuttering. *J. Sp. Hear. Dis.* 17, 316–20.

SHERMAN, D. (1955) Reliability and utility of individual ratings of severity of audible characteristics of stuttering. *J. Sp. Hear. Dis.* 20, 11–16.

SHERMAN, D., YOUNG, M. A. and GOUGH, K. (1958) Comparisons of three measures of stuttering severity. *Proc. Iowa Acad. Sc.* 65, 381–4.

SHULMAN, E. (1955) Factors influencing the variability of stuttering. In *Stuttering in Children and Adults*, ed. W. Johnson, Univ. Minnesota Press, Minneapolis.

SIEGEL, G. M. and HAUGEN, D. (1964) Audience size and variations in stuttering behaviour. *J. Sp. Hear. Res.* 7, 381–8.

SIEGEL, G. M. and MARTIN, R. R. (1965a) Experimental modification of disfluency in normal speakers. *J. Sp. Hear. Res.* 8, 236–44.

SIEGEL, G. M. and MARTIN, R. R. (1965b) Verbal punishment of disfluencies in normal speakers. *J. Sp. Hear. Res.* 8, 245–51.

SIMON, C. T. (1945) Complexity and breakdown in speech situation. *J. Sp. Dis.* 10, 199–203.

SMITH, A. M. (1953) CO_2 therapy in the treatment of stuttering. *Dis. Nerv. System* 14, 243–4.

SMITH, R. G. (1962) A semantic differential for speech correction concepts. *Sp. Monogr.* 29, 32–37.

SNYGG, D. and COMBS, A. W. (1949) *Individual Behaviour: A New Frame of Reference for Psychology*, Harper, New York.

SODERBERG, G. A. (1962) Phonetic influences upon stuttering. *J. Sp. Hear. Res.* 5, 315–20.

SPADINO, E. J. (1941) *Writing and Laterality Characteristics of Stuttering Children*, New York, Columbia Univ., Teachers' College, Contrib. to Educ.

SPENCE, J., WALTON, W. S., MILLER, F. J. W. and COURT, S. D. M. (1954) *A Thousand Families in Newcastle upon Tyne*, Oxford Univ. Press, London.

SPILKA, B. (1954) Relationships between certain aspects of personality and some vocal effects of delayed speech feedback. *J. Sp. Hear. Dis.* 19, 491–503.

SPRIESTERSBACH, D. C. (1940) An exploratory study of the motility of the peripheral oral structures in relation to defective and superior consonant articulation. M.A. thesis, State Univ. Iowa.

SPRIESTERSBACH, D. C. (1951) An objective approach to the investigation of social adjustment of male stutterers. *J. Sp. Hear. Dis.* 16, 250–7.

SSIKORSKI, (1894) *About Stammering* (original in Russian).

STAATS, L. C. JR. (1955) Sense of humor in stutterers and nonstutterers. In *Stuttering in Children and Adults*, ed. W. Johnson, Univ. Minnesota Press, Minneapolis.

STARBUCK, H. B. and STEER, M. D. (1953) The adaptation effect in stuttering speech behaviour. *J. Sp. Hear. Dis.* 18, 252–5.

STARBUCK, H. B. and STEER, M. D. (1954) The adaptation effect in stuttering and its relation to thoracic and abdominal breathing. *J. Sp. Hear. Dis.* 19, 440–9.

STARR, H. E. (1922) The hydrogen ion concentration of the mixed saliva, considered as an index of fatigue and of emotional excitement, and applied to the study of the metabolic etiology of stammering. *Am. J. Psychol.* 33, 394–418.

STARR, H. E. (1928) Psychological commonmitants of higher alveolar carbon dioxide; a psychobiochemical study of the etiology of stammering. *Psychol. Clinic* **17**, 1–12.

STEER, M. D. (1935) A qualitative study of breathing in young stutterers. *Sp. Monogr.* **2**, 1–5.

STEER, M. D. (1937) Symptomatologies of young stutterers. *J. Sp. Dis.* **2**, 3–15.

STEIN, L. (1942) *Speech and Voice: Their Evolution, Pathology and Therapy*, Methuen & Co. Ltd., London.

STEPHENSON, W. A. (1950) A statistical approach to typology. The study of trait universes. *J. Clin. Psychol.* **6**, 26–38.

STEWART, J. L. (1960) The problem of stuttering in certain North American Indian Societies. *J. Sp. Dis.*, Monogr., Suppl., **6**.

ST. ONGE, K. R. (1963) The stuttering syndrome. *J. Sp. Hear. Res.* **6**, 195–7.

ST. ONGE, K. R. and CALVERT, J. J. (1964) Stuttering research. *Quart. J. Sp.* **50**, 159–65.

STRATTON, L. D. (1924) A factor in the etiology of a sub-breathing stammerer: metabolism as indicated by urinary cretine and creatinine. *J. Comp. Psychol.* **4**, 18–27.

STROMSTA, C. P. (1956) A methodology related to the determination of phase angle of bone conducted speech sound energy of stutterers and nonstutterers. Ph.D. diss., Ohio State Univ.

STROTHER, C. (1937) A study of the extent of dyssynergia occurring during the stuttering spasm. *Psychol. Monogr.* **39**, 108–27.

STROTHER, C. R. and KRIEGMAN, L. S. (1943) Diadochokinesis in stutterers and nonstutterers. *J. Sp. Dis.* **8**, 323–5.

STROTHER, C. R. and KRIEGMAN, L. S. (1944) Rhythmokinesis in stutterers and nonstutterers. *J. Sp. Dis.* **9**, 239–44.

SUTTON, S. and CHASE, R. A. (1961) White noise and stuttering. *J. Sp. Hear. Res.* **4**, 72.

TATE, M. W., CULLINAN, W. L. and AHLSTRAND, A. (1961) Measurement of adaptation in stuttering. *J. Sp. Hear. Res.* **4**, 321–39.

TATE, M. W. and CULLINAN, W. L. (1962) Measurement of consistency of stuttering. *J. Sp. Hear. Res.* **5**, 272–83.

TAYLOR, INSUP K. (1966a) What words are stuttered? *Psychol. Bull.* **65**, 233–42.

TAYLOR, INSUP K. (1966b) The properties of stuttered words. *J. Verb. Learn. Verb. Behav.* **5**.

TAYLOR, INSUP K. and TAYLOR, M. M. (1966) Test of predictions from the conflict hypothesis of stuttering (in press). *J. Abn. Psychol.*

TEN CATE, M. J. (1902) Ueber die Untersuchung der Athmungsbewegung bei Sprachfehlern. *Monatschr. f. Sprachheilkunde* **12**, 247.

THOMAS, L. (1951) A personality study of a group of stutterers based on the Minnesota multiphasic personality inventory. M.A. diss., Univ. Oregon.

TIFFANY, W. R. and HANLEY, C. N. (1956) Adaptation to delayed sidetone. *J. Sp. Hear. Dis.* **21**, 164–72.

TRAVIS, L. E. (1927) Studies in stuttering. I. Dysintegration of breathing movements during stuttering. *Arch. Neurol. Psychiat.* **18**, 672–90.

TRAVIS, L. E. (1931) *Speech Pathology*, Appleton, New York.

TRAVIS, L. E. (1934) Dissociation of the homologous muscle in stuttering. *Arch. Neurol. Psychiat.* **31**, 127–33.

TRAVIS, L. E. (1959) *Handbook of Speech Pathology*, Peter Owen, London.

TRAVIS, L. E., JOHNSON, W. and SHOVER, J. (1937) The relations of bilingualism to stuttering, *J. Sp. Dis.* **2**, 185–9.

TRAVIS, L. E. and KNOTT, J. R. (1937) Bilateraly recorded brain potentials from normal speakers and stutterers. *J. Sp. Dis.* **2**, 239.

208   REFERENCES

TRAVIS, L. E., MALAMUD, W. and THAYER, T. R. (1934) The relationship between physical habitus and stuttering. *J. Abn. Soc. Psychol.* **29**, 132–40.

TRAVIS, L. E., TUTTLE, W. W. and COWAN, D. (1936) A study of the heart rate during stuttering. *J. Sp. Dis.* **1**, 21–26.

TROTTER, W. D. (1955) The severity of stuttering during successive readings of the same material. *J. Sp. Hear. Dis.* **20**, 17–25.

TROTTER, W. D. (1956) Relationships between severity of stuttering and word conspicuousness. *J. Sp. Hear. Dis.* **21**, 198–201.

TROTTER, W. D. and KOOLS, J. A. (1955) Listener adaptation to the severity of stuttering. *J. Sp. Hear. Dis.* **20**, 385–7.

TUTHILL, C. E. (1946) A quantitative study of extensional meaning with special reference to stuttering. *Sp. Monogr.* **13**, 81–98.

VAN DUSEN, C. R. (1939) A laterality study of nonstutterers and stutterers. *J. Sp. Dis.* **4**, 261–5.

VAN RIPER, C. (1936) Study of the thoracic breathing of stutterers during expectancy and occurrence of stuttering spasms. *J. Sp. Dis.* **1**, 61–72.

VAN RIPER, C. (1937) The effects of penalty upon the frequency of stuttering spasms. *J. Genet. Psychol.* **50**, 193–5.

VAN RIPER, C. (1954) *Speech Correction: Principles and Methods*, 3rd ed., Prentice-Hall.

VAN RIPER, C. and HULL, C. J. (1955) The quantitative measurement of the effect of certain situations on stuttering. In *Stuttering in Children and Adults*, ed. W. Johnson, Univ. Minnesota Press, Minneapolis.

VAN RIPER, C. and MILISEN, R. L. (1939) A study of the predicted duration of the stutterers' blocks as related to their actual duration. *J. Sp. Dis.* **4**, 339–45.

VERNON, P. E. (1964) *Personality Assessment*, Methuen, London.

VOELKER, C. H. (1944) A preliminary investigation for a normative study of fluency: a clinical index to the severity of stuttering. *Am. J. Orthopsychiat.* **14**, 285–94.

WADA, J. and RASMUSSEN, T. (1960) Intracarotid injection of sodium amytal for the lateralization of cerebral speech dominance. Experimental and clinical observations. *J. Neurosurg.* **17**, 266–82.

WALLEN, V. (1959) A Q-technique study of self-concepts of adolescent stutterers and nonstutterers. Doct. diss., Boston Univ.

WALNUT, A. (1954) A personality inventory item analysis of individuals who stutter and individuals who have other handicaps. *J. Sp. Hear. Dis.* **19**, 220–7.

WENDAHL, R. W. and COLE, JANE (1961) Identification of stuttering during relatively fluent speech. *J. Sp. Hear. Res.* **4**, 281–6.

WEPMAN, J. M. (1939) Familial incidence in stammering. *J. Sp. Dis.* **4**, 199–204.

WEST, R. (1929) A neurological test for stutterers. *J. Neurol. Psychopathol.* **10**, 114–23.

WEST, R. (1958) An agnostic's speculations about stuttering. In *Stuttering: A Symposium*, ed. J. Eisenson, Harper, New York.

WEST, R., NELSON, S. and BERRY, M. (1939) The heredity of stuttering. *Quart. J. Sp.* **25**, 23–30.

WESTPHAL, G. (1933) An experimental study of certain motor abilities of stutterers. *Child Develop.* **4**, 214–21.

WILLIAMS, D. (1955) Masseter muscle action potentials in stuttered and non-stuttered speech. *J. Sp. Hear. Dis.* **20**, 242–61.

WILLIAMS, D. E. and KENT, LOUISE R. (1958) Listener evaluations of speech interruptions. *J. Sp. Hear. Res.* **1**, 124–31.

WILLIAMS, D. E., WARK, MICHELLE and MINIFIE, F. D. (1963) Ratings of stuttering by audio, visual and audiovisual cues. *J. Sp. Hear. Res.* **6**, 91–100.

209

WILSON, D. M. (1951) A study of the personalities of stuttering children and their parents as revealed through projective tests. *Sp. Monogr.* **18**, 133.

WINCHESTER, R. A., GIBBONS, E. W. and KREBS, D. F. (1959) Adaptation to sustained delayed sidetone. *J. Sp. Hear. Dis.* **24**, 25–28.

WINGATE, M. E. (1959) Calling attention to stuttering. *J. Sp. Hear. Res.* **2**, 326–35.

WINGATE, M. E. (1962a) Evaluation of stuttering. Part I. Speech characteristics of young children. *J. Sp. Hear. Dis.* **27**, No. 2, 106–15.

WINGATE, M. E. (1962b) Evaluation and stuttering. Part II. Environmental stress and critical appraisal of speech. *J. Sp. Hear. Dis.* **27**, No. 3, 244–57.

WINGATE, M. E. (1962c) Evaluation and stuttering. Part III. Identification of stuttering and the use of a label. *J. Sp. Hear. Dis.* **27**, No. 4, 368–77.

WINGATE, M. E. (1964) A standard definition of stuttering. *J. Sp. Hear. Dis.* **29**, 484–9.

WINGATE, M. E. (1965) A reply. *J. Sp. Hear. Dis.* **30**, 200–2.

WINKELMAN, N. W. JR. (1954) Chlorpromazine in the treatment of neuropsychiatric disorders. *J. Am. Med. Assoc.* **155**, 18–21.

WISCHNER, G. J. (1947) Stuttering behaviour and learning: a program of research. Ph.D. diss., Univ. Iowa.

WISCHNER, G. J. (1948) An experimental approach to stuttering as learned behaviour. *Am. Psychologist*, **3**, 278–9.

WISCHNER, G. J. (1950) Stuttering behaviour and learning: a preliminary theoretical formulation. *J. Sp. Hear. Dis.* **15**, 324–35.

WISCHNER, G. J. (1952) An experimental approach to expectancy and anxiety in stuttering behaviour. *J. Sp. Hear. Dis.* **17**, 139–54.

WOHL, M. T. (1951) Incidence of speech defects in the population. *Speech* **15**, 13.

WOOLF, G. (1965) A definition in search of data and a theory. *J. Sp. Hear. Dis.* **30**, 199–200.

WYLIE, R. C. (1961) *The Self-Concept: A Critical Survey of Pertinent Research Literature*, Univ. Nebraska Press, Lincoln, Nebraska.

YATES, A. J. (1963) Delayed auditory feedback. *Psychol. Bull.* **60**, 213–32.

YOUNG, M. A. (1961) Predicting ratings of severity of stuttering. *J. Sp. Hear. Dis.*, Monogr. Suppl., **7**, 31–54.

YOUNG, M. A. (1965) Audience size, perceived situational difficulty, and stuttering frequency. *J. Sp. Hear. Res.* **8**, 401–7.

YOUNG, M. A. and PRATHER, E. M. (1962) Measuring severity of stuttering using short segments of speech. *J. Sp. Hear. Res.* **5**, 256–62.

ZELEN, S. L., SHEEHAN, J. G. and BUGENTAL, J. F. T. (1954) Self-perceptions in stuttering. *J. Clin. Psychol.* **10**, 70–72.

ZIPF, G. K. (1949) *Human Behaviour and the Principle of Least Effort*, Addison-Wesley, Cambridge, Mass.

AUTHOR INDEX

SUBJECT INDEX

Achievement motivation 112
Adaptation effect 136–61
  and age 147, 149
  and anxiety level 120, 148, 154
  and anxiety reduction 66
  and breathing patterns 100
  and in children 35
  and definition 136
  and delayed auditory feedback 59,
    167, 168
  and drugs 93
  and expectancy 68, 127–8, 147, 148,
    149
  and experimental extinction 136,
    155
  and fatigue 140
  and the listener 43, 149–54
  and methods of eliciting speech 137
  and the nonstutterer 149–54, 159
  and prediction 151, 153, 154, 159
  and prognosis 137, 147, 154–5,
    159
  and propositionality 63, 158
  and punishment 190
  and reactive inhibition 157
  and relapse 175
  and reliability 146–7, 159
  and scoring 140, 146, 159
  and severity of stuttering 154
  and silent reading 156
  and situational anxiety 67
  and spontaneous recovery 160–2
  and spontaneous speech 137–9, 159
  and subgroups of stutterers 151,
    154, 159
  and syntax 142
  and theories of 155–9
  and time intervals between readings
    142–3, 159, 160, 161
  and transfer 137, 149
  and transition probability 135
  and treatment 137, 147, 154–5, 159,
    160
  and type and size of audience 142,
    143–6

  and type of material 67, 93, 139–42,
    159
  and type of situation 142, 143–6
  and typical experimental situation
    139
  and verbal conditioning 182
  and word avoidance 138–9
Adrenalin 87
Aetiology 3, 68, 79, 183, 184
  and metabolism 24, 90
  and reinforcement theory 183–5
  and stress 16
  theories of
    anatomical 105
    neurological 24, 106, 141, 163
    physiological 24, 105, 106, 141
    psychological 24, 60, 105
Age 15–20, 73
  and anxiety level 120
  and development of stuttering 35
  and differences 5, 13
  and incidence 12
  and motor symptomatology 10
  and onset 18, 98
  and sex ratio 23
Aggression 75, 110, 112, 121
Allergic reaction 87, 103
Anticipation 65, 66, 67, 68, 73
Anti-social behaviour 27
Anxiety
  general 120–1
  situational 66, 67, 113, 120, 122,
    144
  specific word 66, 67, 120, 141, 142,
    144
Anxiety level 25, 27, 66, 73, 76, 115,
    122, 124, 159, 178, 188
  and adaptation 63, 120, 148, 154
  and age 120
  and blocking 64
  and EEG correlates 97
  and parents 27, 70
  and perseveration 64
  and severity of stuttering 151
  and tranquillizers 94, 95, 96